DATE DUE

AUG 03 1993			
APR 26 1994			

PRACTICAL OBSTETRICAL ULTRASOUND

John W. Seeds, M.D.
Assistant Professor
Department of Obstetrics and Gynecology
Division of Maternal and Fetal Medicine
University of North Carolina School of Medicine
Chapel Hill, North Carolina

Robert C. Cefalo, M.D., Ph.D.
Professor
Department of Obstetrics and Gynecology
Division of Maternal and Fetal Medicine
University of North Carolina School of Medicine
Chapel Hill, North Carolina

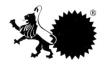

AN ASPEN PUBLICATION®
Aspen Publishers, Inc.
Rockville, Maryland
Royal Tunbridge Wells
1986

Library of Congress Cataloging in Publication Data

Seeds, John W.
Practical obstetrical ultrasound.

"An Aspen publication."
Includes bibliographies and index.
1. Ultrasonics in obstetrics. I. Cefalo, Robert C.
II. Title. [DNLM: 1. Pregnancy Complications —
diagnosis. 2. Prenatal Diagnosis — methods.
3. Ultrasonic Diagnosis — in pregnancy. WQ 209 S451p]
RG527.5.U48S44   1986   618.2'07543   85-31556
ISBN: 0-87189-273-1

Editorial Services: M. Eileen Higgins

Library of Congress Catalog Card Number: 85-31556
ISBN: 0-87189-273-1

Printed in the United States of America

1   2   3   4   5

To the people of North Carolina
Whose experiences with ultrasound
Provide the basis for
Most of the illustrations
In this book

I would like to thank and acknowledge
Mickey Senkarik, M.S., A.M.I.,
the artist who created this book's line drawings.

Table of Contents

Foreword

Most members of the medical community, and especially those who practice obstetrics and gynecology, must be knowledgeable in the use of ultrasound. Twenty years ago, ultrasound was only a promising technique that had potential for obstetrical applications. Its safety was not yet known, but it appeared on theoretical grounds to offer a modality for diagnosis that would be harmless to both the mother and fetus during pregnancy. As time progressed, this safety seemed to prove true.

Despite numerous studies to evaluate the possible harmful effects of ultrasound energy, no clinically harmful effects have been identified in those patients and their children who have been exposed to ultrasound beams from a variety of sources under different conditions. While it is impossible to provide an absolute guarantee of the safety of diagnostic ultrasound, those working in the field are growing more confident as time passes.

With this increasing confidence comes broader applicability and more generalized use of clinical ultrasound. Ultrasound is now a realistic consideration for the clinical practitioner in the office as well as within hospitals and radiology units. Furthermore, there has been striking technological progress in the development of medical ultrasound equipment, and this progress has been rapid and impressive.

The original clinical ultrasound consisted of a black and white image that could be used in the A mode, to demonstrate interface surfaces, and in the B mode, to generate a simple black and white image. We now have the capability to do real-time gray-scale, sector scanning, M mode, flow studies, and, in the near future, color-enhanced sonographic scanning. The improvements in resolution and shading have taken us to the point of being able to evaluate fetal eye movements and study the fetal lens in utero. This enormous technical capability has permitted us to seek ever more precise and accurate diagnoses. With the availability of small portable real-time units and sector scanners, direct observation of the fetus while performing fetal surgical procedures under ultrasound guidance is a reality today.

Thus, ultrasound is an important part of the current clinical and research armamentarium in obstetrics and gynecology. As with most clinical subjects, skill is acquired by practical experience, and only a very special textbook is helpful. *Practical Obstetrical Ultrasound* is such a book. It is designed specifically for the clinical practitioner and is both concise and practical. In that it also offers direct guidance, it is, in fact, a how-to-do-it book. Anyone learning to use clinical ultrasound for the first time will find the text clear and the description of technique very easy to follow. More experienced sonographers will benefit from the descriptive paragraphs and the superb photographs illustrating the points made by the text. In addition, there are key references at the end of each chapter that permit in-depth study of the various topics covered.

The use of ultrasound for a variety of purposes in obstetrics and gynecology seems firmly established. All of us within this specialty must be familiar with the techniques that will be beneficial to our patients. In addition, we are held responsible by society for failure to diagnose those things that may be demonstrable by sonographic techniques. Finally, physicians are perpetual students. As new ideas come along and technologies become available to clinical practitioners, we must continue to learn and to put these new ideas and technologies into use in our daily practice.

In western Europe, ultrasound is a routine part of every obstetrical patient's care. While this has not become the case in the United States yet, it is foreseeable that it will in the near future as the public begins to demand every possible diagnostic advantage in the care of pregnant women.

While the most recent consensus conference sponsored by the National Institutes of Health did not endorse routine ultrasound in pregnancy, the indications for its use are so broadly stated that it is a semantic distinction rather than a real one. Eventually, if we are to practice the best quality of obstetrical care, ultrasound screening will become routine. This will enhance our capability to offer an early diagnosis of certain congenital anomalies. It also will oblige us to make a diagnosis in those few unfortunate cases where there has been no reason to suspect it. Thus, a skilled ultrasonographic examination will become as much a part of obstetrical care as a skilled interpretation of a chest x-ray is a part of the care rendered by the general internist. While this may seem unrealistic now, it is well within the realm of possibility. And in the not so very distant future.

It seems likely that whatever the future holds for ultrasound in the United States, we need to have a very thorough knowledge of its clinical use and be able to interpret it for our patients. Dr. Seeds and Dr. Cefalo have given us a practical clinical guide to set us on that forward path.

Bruce K. Young, M.D.
Director of Maternal and Fetal Medicine
New York University Medical Center

Preface

Most of the textbooks on obstetrical ultrasound are excellent documentary reviews of the technology and the applications of diagnostic ultrasound in pregnancy. In many cases, however, readers searching for an instructional experience may not be satisfied with extensive discussions of physics or obscure illustrations with variable visual clarity derived from diverse equipment. Our objective in *Practical Obstetrical Ultrasound* is to provide an introduction to this imaging technique and also to examine the latest methodologies and clinical applications. An instructional approach is used and illustrations are derived from contemporary realtime equipment. Sonograms are complemented when necessary by simple line drawings. Examples and problems are provided when appropriate to illustrate selected techniques.

It is no more necessary for the clinician to master the finite detail of sonic physics in order to perform quality imaging than it is necessary for every driver of an automobile with an automatic transmission to appreciate the details of hydraulic mechanics. However, there must be a minimal understanding of the physical behavior of ultrasound and a comprehension of the interactions between this type of energy and biological tissue. This information forms a basis for considerations of safety, as well as for the rational evaluation of various available systems. Such a conceptual understanding of the principles of ultrasound may be achieved easily and comfortably without complex mathematical formulae.

Ultrasound has been a revolutionary development in clinical obstetrics that has increased the quantity and quality of information available to the clinician active in the management of pregnancy. Sonography may be used to confirm or establish gestational age, establish fetal viability, assess the quality of fetal growth and fetal condition, localize the placenta, guide invasive procedures, and diagnose fetal malformations. Clinical perspectives are presented along with the techniques in those chapters devoted to fetal growth retardation, gestational age assignment, and prenatal diagnosis.

The most deceptive aspect of obstetrical ultrasound is the apparent ease with which it may be performed. The freehand transducer of contemporary realtime ultrasound equipment offers unlimited flexibility in creating images of the uterine contents. Ultrasound equipment is freely available. There is the danger, however, that clinical errors might result from well-intentioned but poorly or incompletely performed ultrasound examinations. Accurate and sensitive sonography requires patience, experience, and a devotion to detail and completeness. The quality of referral and backup resources and the availability of instructional workshops with hands-on teaching are also important. Clinicians cannot base clinical management on their own ultrasound data until an appropriate level of confidence has been achieved.

Our instruction will begin with a brief review of those principles of the physical properties of sound that will allow proper interpretation of both the images produced and the various configurations of available equipment. Then, after an examination of normal ultrasonic fetal anatomy, gestational dating methods are reviewed. A discussion of the use of ultrasound in the assessment of the quality of fetal growth and fetal well-being includes clinical guidelines for the interpretation of ultrasonic data. In later chapters we illustrate certain fetal malformations that might be detected with ultrasound. Finally, the logistics of office-based ultrasound are discussed, along with user liability in an office setting.

Throughout these pages we endeavor to use simplified language and uncluttered illustrations. When necessary, words peculiar to ultrasound imaging are defined and/or illustrated. The suggested readings are intended to give those readers interested in further information access to important articles relevant to a particular discussion. Reference tables and charts are chosen for their practical clinical value and are often modified to simplify their use. When gestational age is referred to, it is measured from last menstrual period, not conception. The duration of normal pregnancy is, therefore, assumed to be 40 weeks.

So, then, don't be intimidated or afraid to begin exploring this exciting new clinical tool called ultrasound.

J.W.S.

R.C.C.

PRACTICAL OBSTETRICAL ULTRASOUND

Chapter 1

The Necessary Minimal Physics and A Look at Safety

A basic appreciation of the physical properties of sound energy is important for the sonographer or sonologist to interpret properly the images and artifacts often seen during scanning. In this chapter we will consider conceptual principles of sound and sound imaging systems and briefly review considerations of human safety.

SOUND

Sound is a form of kinetic energy rapidly propagated away from the source through any mass-containing substance. Sound consists of moving phases of higher than normal pressure (density) alternating with intervening phases of lower than normal pressure (density). These pressure phases are arranged in planes arrayed across the axis of their propagation (Fig 1-1). Sound passage actually produces a physical oscillation or agitation of the molecules of the medium with molecular movement forward and back in the direction of the axis of propagation.

Such alternate planar pressure phases (sound) can be produced by the oscillating movement of a surface in contact with the medium repetitively compressing the adjacent surface of the medium. Since the natural intermolecular electromagnetic forces of any substance tend to resist deformation, any transient pressure or density change will be passed by these forces from one spatial zone to the next in a direction away from the source. Although sound really comprises planar pressure pulses, not waves, it may be graphically described using a waveform to show both the frequency and the amplitude of pressure changes (see Fig 1-1).

Sound may be described by its frequency, which is indicated in complete cycles per second, or cps (1 cps = 1 hertz). Any sound beam with a frequency over 20,000 hertz (abbreviated Hz) is above the range of the human ear, and such high frequency sound is called ultrasound. In medical

3

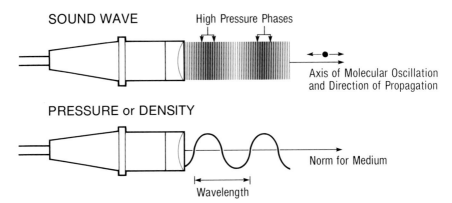

SOUND WAVE High Pressure Phases

Axis of Molecular Oscillation and Direction of Propagation

PRESSURE or DENSITY

Norm for Medium

Wavelength

Fig 1-1. Sound waves. Sound waves are actually high pressure phases moving away from the source that produce molecular agitation in the transmission medium. The upper drawing illustrates the high pressure or high density phases, as well as the molecular movement forward and back in the same axis as the direction of propagation. The lower drawing illustrates the same concept in a graphic form.

applications, frequencies in the range of 1 to 10 million Hz or 1 to 10 megahertz (abbreviated MHz) are often used. The frequencies most often used in obstetrical applications are 2.5 to 3.5 MHz (2.5 to 3.5 million cycles or complete pressure phase oscillations per second).

The source of sound of such high frequencies is the piezoelectric crystal. Piezoelectric crystals may be naturally occurring (quartz is one) or synthetic. They have the property of changing their shape when stimulated by a transient voltage potential (Fig 1-2). When exposed to an almost instantaneous electric stimulus, a crystal continues to vibrate with a frequency unique to the crystalline structure unless damped. Conversely, piezoelectric crystals generate a tiny electric signal when squeezed or stretched as they would be if in the path of a sound beam composed of intermittent pressure peaks and valleys. The tiny electric signals generated may be detected and catalogued electronically. Piezoelectric crystals are, therefore, capable not only of producing very high frequency sound in response to sequenced pulses of voltage potential but also of detecting high frequency sound. Thin wafers of piezoelectric crystal may be mounted in the surface of small devices called transducers that transform electric signals into sound pulses and sound pulses back into electric signals. The length of each sound pulse generated is determined by the timing of the voltage stimulus and by the design of special damping systems constructed to limit the duration of vibration. The

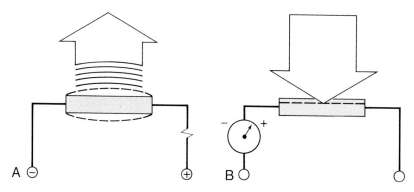

Fig 1-2. Piezoelectric crystal. (*A*) A piezoelectric crystal is shown to change its shape in response to an electric pulse. This change in shape produces alternate phases of high and low pressure in any adjacent transmission medium and, therefore, constitutes a source for sound waves. (*B*) The piezoelectric crystal is also shown to be a detector of sound waves as it generates a slight electric potential when compressed as if in the path of a sound beam of alternate high and low pressure phases.

pulse length may be limited to as little as one complete wavelength. The planar shape of the pressure phases (sound wave) is at first similar to the surface shape of the transducer surface, but eventually this fidelity to crystal shape deteriorates and is lost (Fig 1-3).

Sound travels through substances at a speed influenced by the frequency of the sound and by the stiffness or resistance to molecular movement of the

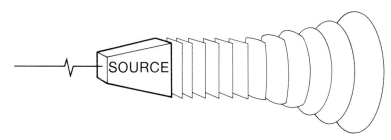

Fig 1-3. Divergence. The phases of high and low pressure traveling away from the source of agitation will maintain reasonable fidelity to the source until divergence causes the pressure phases gradually to become concentric spheres.

tissue (acoustical impedance). The speed of sound in soft tissue is assumed by convention to average 1540 meters per second. The actual speed for specific tissues varies above or below 1540 meters per second relative to the acoustical impedance, but this average is used as the basis for most contemporary imaging systems. Sound will travel through a substance until all of its energy is dissipated. The energy level or intensity of a sound beam may be described by the amplitude of the corresponding sine wave. Dissipation of the energy of a sound beam (attenuation) occurs as a function of loss to heat, loss by reflection or scatter, and loss due to divergence. Heat is produced overcoming the inherent molecular resistance to movement (molecular inertia) of the transmission medium. The amount of heat produced is inversely related to the stiffness of the substance or tissue. This attenuation results in a loss of amplitude, not a change of frequency or of wavelength. The maximum distance of travel (depth of penetration in the case of soft tissue imaging systems) is dependent both on the frequency of the beam and the density or rigidity of the tissue, as well as on the number of surfaces encountered that produce reflections. The higher the frequency, the greater is the loss of amplitude to heat per centimeter of travel. A 5-MHz sound beam will not penetrate soft tissue as deeply as a 2.5-MHz sound beam of comparable initial intensity (amplitude).

Reflection of sound energy in the form of echos also leads to gradual loss of intensity of the primary beam. When a sound pulse beam encounters a surface or interface between two tissues of differing acoustical impedance (stiffness or rigidity), reflection of a portion of the energy occurs and an echo is produced. Such an echo is of the same wavelength as the primary sound pulse unless the surface is moving. The amplitude of the echo is subtracted from the transmitted primary pulse (Fig 1-4). The amplitude of the reflected echo is determined by the difference in stiffness between the two tissues (acoustical impedance difference). The greater the impedance difference, the greater is the amplitude of the echo and the weaker is the primary pulse beam transmitted through the interface or surface.

If the primary pulse beam is perpendicular to the surface, the echo will travel back to the source and may be detected. The information from such echos may then contribute to the composition of an image. If the angle of incidence is not 90°, the echo will be reflected at an equal angle and lost as scatter. Scatter also attenuates the primary beam but contributes nothing to an image.

Divergence is a process that also gradually decreases the intensity of any radiant energy form as it travels away from the source. The edges of a discrete radiant waveform tend to turn away from the axis of the primary beam, spreading the energy of the beam over a greater area, decreasing the amplitude (Fig 1-5). The intensity or amplitude remains greatest at the center of such a beam, decreasing gradually toward the boundaries.

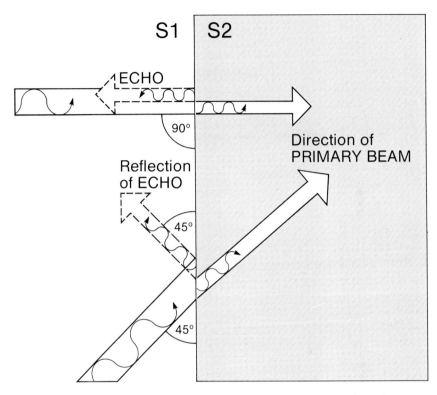

Fig 1-4. Reflections. When sound pulses encounter a surface between two tissues (S1 and S2) of different stiffness, a portion of the sound energy is reflected, producing an echo. If the incident sound pulse is at a right angle to the surface, the reflected pulse travels back in the direction of the incident beam, as in the upper drawing. If the incident sound pulse is at any other angle, the angle of reflection equals the angle of incidence, as illustrated in the lower drawing. In both cases, the amplitude or intensity of the echo is subtracted from the amplitude or intensity of the transmitted beam.

ECHOS AND IMAGES

Echos are the basis of the ultrasound image. Since the average speed of sound in soft tissue may be set, the time of generation and the time of echo arrival establish the depth (range) of an echo-producing surface. A single ultrasound crystal/transducer may in this way be used to measure simple linear distance (Fig 1-6). If a computer is set to record and display on a

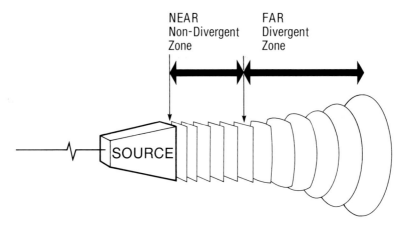

Fig 1-5. The near zone. Lateral resolution is optimized when the anatomy of interest is within the near nondivergent zone of a sound beam. When the anatomy of interest occupies a depth within the far divergent zone, resolution is hampered.

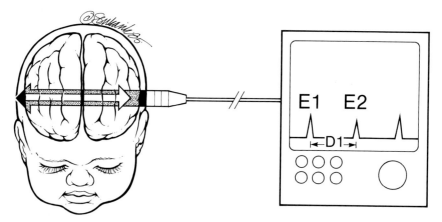

Fig 1-6. A-mode. If an oscilloscope screen is calibrated to the speed of sound and the arrival time of reflected echos, then linear distance may be measured as illustrated here. E1 indicates the deflection of the baseline (amplitude modulation) representing the arrival of the echo from the proximal skull table of this infant's head. E2 indicates an echo from the midline and, therefore, D1 may be adjusted to represent the distance between the skull table and the midline. This application of a single ultrasound beam to measure linear distance is called A-mode.

screen in two dimensions many bits of this sort of linear data, then a single transducer (crystal) may be moved over the surface of a subject in a single plane, and it is possible to produce a composite image of cross-sectional anatomy from these echos (Fig 1-7). The system remains aware of the spatial location of the transducer as it is moved across the patient by the use of stereotactic joints of an articulated arm. This sort of machine could not show realtime movement. In fact, any movement would blur the image by changing the relative spatial location of the various tissue surfaces during the composition of the image.

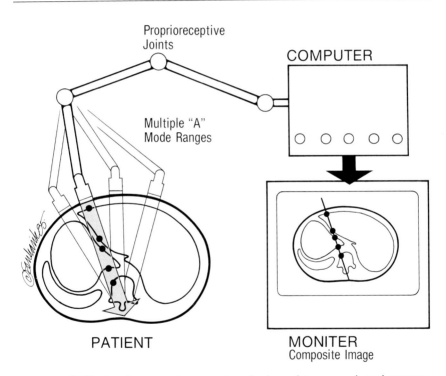

Proprioreceptive
Joints

COMPUTER

Multiple "A"
Mode Ranges

PATIENT

MONITER
Composite Image

Fig 1-7. B-Mode. A computer may be designed to record and remember the distance from the transducer surface of echos derived from a series of single beam pulses. A composite image of soft tissue anatomy within a single plane may then be constructed in two dimensions using this information. In this case, the brightness of a specific spot on the display screen is modulated with regard to the presence or absence of an echo from that location.

If a series of crystal elements were aligned within a single transducer housing and their location relative to one another fixed, the relative locations of tissue surfaces producing echos heard by the various crystals would also be fixed. A two-dimensional image could then be composed from the echos from the field of scan lines without the need for any articulated attachment to the console computer. This is the concept of the *linear array realtime ultrasound machine*. Usually several adjacent elements are activated as a team, with successive overlapping teams activated sequentially (Fig 1-8). Elements along the entire length of the transducer are activated in turn repetitively and rapidly. This process allows almost continuous renewal of the anatomical information on the display screen and thus enables the depiction of movement in realtime. Specific machines vary in the total

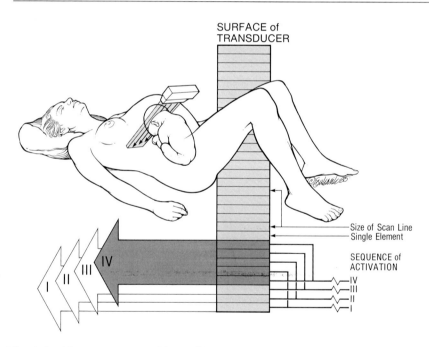

Fig 1-8. Linear array realtime. This composite illustration depicts the surface of a linear array realtime transducer and shows the activation of teams of individual crystal elements along the face of the transducer. In addition, the field of view originating from such a transducer is illustrated on the drawing of the fetus. In this particular example, all members of the team of transducers are being activated synchronously.

number of elements within their transducer, in the exact composition of the "teams," and also in the exact electronic sequencing.

Mechanical sector scanners use one or more crystal elements that either oscillate within the transducer or rotate within it on a shaft. These machines produce sound pulses and listen for echos in 60° to 90° arcs, or sectors, providing a wedge-shaped field of view (Fig 1-9). The small contact area required is a major advantage in certain applications.

Gray scaling is the arbitrary adjustment of the brightness of a display point on the display screen in proportion to the intensity of the echo. Gray scaling may be exactly proportional, with the brightness of the screen dot exactly and directly related to the strength of the echo, or there may be variable emphasis using an arbitrary weighting system. The number of shades of gray varies from 16 to 64. Gray scaling is designed to enhance the operator's ability to discriminate tissue textures. However, various gray scale emphasis weighting systems may be variably appealing to an individual eye and lead to system selection based not on absolute resolving power but on image appearance. Time delay adjustment (*automatic time gain*) is performed before gray scaling and is automatic in most systems. Automatic

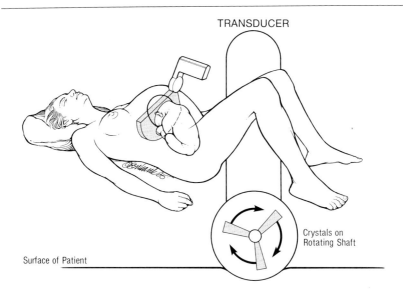

TRANSDUCER

Crystals on Rotating Shaft

Surface of Patient

Fig 1-9. Mechanical sector. This particular example of a sector scanner depicts three crystal elements attached to a rotating shaft in contact with the patient's abdominal wall. The crystal elements are activated within a 90° arc, or sector, and produce a wedge-shaped field of view.

time gain simply amplifies the intensity of echos in proportion to the time delay between generation of the primary pulse and arrival of the echo. This amplification compensates for the expected average attenuation loss and keeps the image intensity uniform throughout the field of view. Most systems allow manual adjustment of gain at selected depths to compensate for individual differences.

RESOLUTION

The ability to discriminate one point as discrete from another is called *resolution*. Ultrasonic imaging equipment is concerned with the ability to resolve two-dimensional anatomical detail, but if sonographic images are reduced to individual scan lines, sharpness is really a matter of the ability to discriminate between discrete "points." *Lateral resolution* describes the ability of an imaging system to resolve two points lying in a plane perpendicular to the direction of propagation of the beam (two points aligned with the x-axis of the display screen) (Fig 1-10). Lateral resolving power is directly related to the width of the sound beam (beam width) at the level of the points in question. The narrowest beam width at the depth of interest determines the quality of the image in this dimension at that depth. Beam width varies with distance from the source and is a function of divergence. Close to the source, the beam width remains similar to crystal width. The

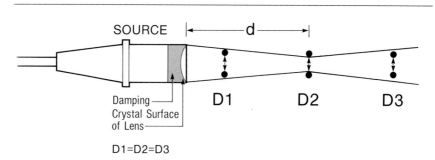

D1=D2=D3

Fig 1-10. Fixed focus. Focusing material built into the surface of a single element transducer or manufacturing the shape of the crystal in a manner that results in a converging ultrasound beam will result in maximum lateral resolution at a specified depth (d). In this illustration, all three pairs of points are an equal distance apart. However, clear resolution of the two points at depth two (D2) will be accomplished because of minimum beam width at that depth.

larger the crystal, the farther from the source the beam travels before significant divergence occurs. At some depth from any transducer, divergence will invariably occur and lateral resolution will deteriorate. Points will appear as streaks across the screen when lateral resolution is lost.

The wider the crystal, the longer is the near nondivergent "narrow" zone, but with a wider crystal, the wider primary beam produces a direct loss of lateral resolving power. In the case of linear array realtime machines, as we have seen, the aligned elements are pulsed in groups of four or five at a time. That is, for example, crystals number one through four, then numbers two through five, and so on (see Fig 1-8). In terms of divergence, the sound pulses from a team act as if they were from one crystal element of the same overall size as the whole group. This design provides an individual beam with a nondivergent zone that is longer than would be expected from an individual crystal because it is proportional to the width of the team. The resolving power of such a system, however, can be closer to that expected from a single element owing to the overlapping of teams on a single-element basis.

If the activation of the outermost members of a team of crystals occurs slightly before the central members, the sound beam is forced inward or focused (Fig 1-11). The beam will narrow to a minimum at a depth governed by the degree of asynchrony of activation. The sound pulses will diverge beyond that point. Most contemporary systems allow the user to alter the sequence delay and, therefore, alter the depth of maximum lateral resolution.

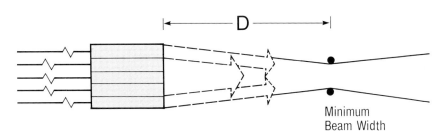

Minimum
Beam Width

Fig 1-11. Electronic focusing. If the electronic activation of the outside members of any phased team occurs slightly before the activation of the central elements, the beam from this source will be forced inward, essentially resulting in a focusing of the beam to a minimum beam width at a given depth (D), which relates to the degree of asynchrony in the activation of the elements. This form of electronic focusing may be varied by the operator.

Beam width is also focused by most linear array systems in the third dimension (z-axis), perpendicular to the plane of the scan tomogram. The beam width in this direction affects the thickness of the slice. Usually the beam is focused through crystal curvature or focusing lenses that are not variable after manufacture. The depth of minimum beam width in this case is permanent and is chosen to coincide with likely anatomy of interest (Fig 1-12).

Axial resolution describes the power of a system to discriminate or resolve as separate two points or surfaces lying on a line in the axis of propagation of the sound beam and analogous to anatomy aligned with the y-axis of the display (Fig 1-13). Axial resolution is related to pulse length. The pulse length is determined by the design of the damping material, and in most systems a crystal is active for about a microsecond every millisecond, or 0.1% of any given time interval. The shorter the pulse length, the greater is the axial resolution. Pulse length is limited by wavelength. The shorter the wavelength (higher frequencies), the shorter may be the pulse. However, higher frequencies also result in greater tissue attenuation and

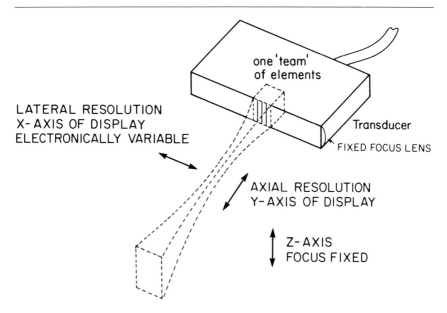

Fig 1-12. Combined focus. The combined effect of a built-in fixed focusing lens system and an electronically variable focusing system is to produce a single scan line with a minimum beam width in both the lateral or x-axis of display, as well as perpendicular to the plane of the tomogram.

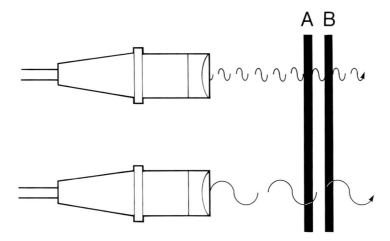

Fig 1-13. Axial resolution. The ability to discriminate between tissue surface (A) and tissue surface (B) depends on the pulse length. The upper ultrasound beam with the short pulse length (higher frequency) will be better able to discriminate these tissue planes than the lower ultrasound transducer of longer wavelength, longer pulse length, and lower frequency.

reduced penetration. Frequency choice is, therefore, a compromise between resolution and penetration and depends on the typical depth of targeted organs. In obstetrics, 2.5 and 3.5 MHz are the most popular frequencies. Attenuation may be overcome to some extent in the case of higher frequencies by increasing the power of the primary beam, but this would necessarily also increase heat deposition, and the increase in image clarity is rarely profound.

EQUIPMENT CATEGORIES

Contact Gray Scale

Also known as B-scan, compound scanner, contact scanner, or static B-scan, this machine uses a single transducer on a stereotactic articulated arm to compose a static image from the integrated echo points accumulated from multiple individual pulse beams produced as the transducer is passed over the patient in a single plane. *Advantages:* The field of view is capable of encompassing the entire third trimester uterus. There is very good lateral resolution of deep tissues and good penetration (Fig 1-14). *Disadvantages:* The cost is high. It is immobile and very large and cannot demonstrate dynamic movement.

Sector Realtime

One crystal oscillates or multiple elements rotate within the transducer housing. Sound energy is pulsed in a 60° to 90° arc from the face of the transducer, producing a wedge-shaped field of view. Sector scanners show movement in realtime (Fig 1-15). *Advantages:* The small contact area required allows imaging of the newborn brain through a fontanelle or imaging of deep pelvic anatomy such as ovarian follicles from a limited suprapubic access area. It is more affordable than static machines and usually is quite mobile. Sector transducers are easily covered with sterile plastic bags for intraoperative applications. *Disadvantages:* The narrow near

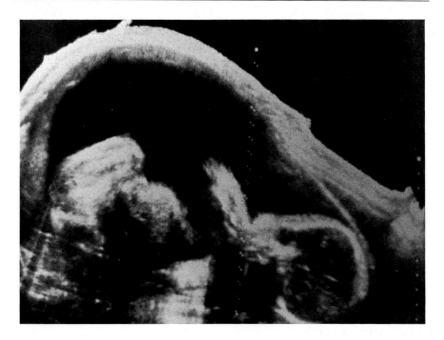

Fig 1-14. Contact gray scale. This sonogram was derived from a compound gray scale ultrasound machine. It is a machine capable of including the entire third trimester in a single field of view. Illustrated here is a fetus of 34 weeks' gestation with polyhydramnios, which appears black in this sonogram.

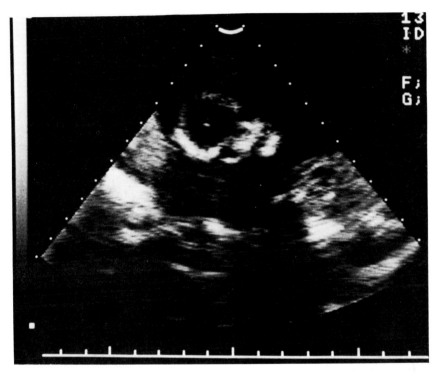

Fig 1-15. Sector scanner. The mechanical sector realtime machine produces a field of view that is wedge shaped owing to the activation of the crystals only within a 60° to 90° arc. The field of view at the upper portion of this sonogram is limited in its capacity. The far field, which is wider, is somewhat imperfect in its resolution. Seen here are the anterior facial features of a fetus at 17 weeks' gestation.

field of view limits this machine's usefulness in the second half of pregnancy. There is greater geometric distortion than linear array and greater loss of clarity in the far field.

Linear Array Realtime

Multiple, fixed, focused elements are aligned and pulsed in phases to produce a rectangular field of view with realtime movement (Fig 1-16). *Advantages:* There is a larger near field than sector and less geometric distortion in the far field. It is more affordable than static machines and

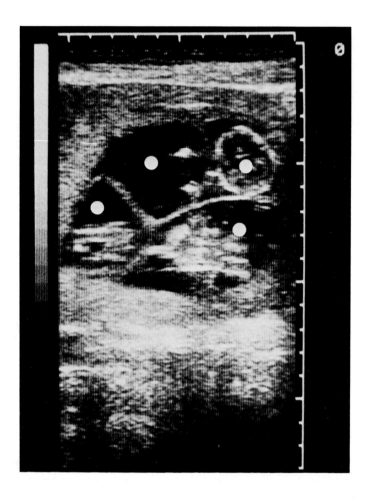

Fig 1-16. Linear array realtime. The linear array realtime ultrasound machine produces a rectangular field of view. The sharpness or clarity of the near field (upper portion of the scan) is superior to what is seen in the far field. However, the capacity does not change. Illustrated here is an early pregnancy with quadruplets. Each white dot appears within a separate gestational sac. In the gestational sac at the upper right the sonogram illustrates an approximately appropriate plane for a biparietal diameter for that particular fetus.

usually is quite mobile. *Disadvantages:* The size of the transducer limits applications that involve limited contact area.

SAFETY CONSIDERATIONS

Sound passing through tissue deposits heat. The amount of heat depends on the intensity (amplitude) of the sound beam and varies with frequency and tissue impedance (stiffness). Intensity may be expressed as watts per square centimeter (W/cm^2), or milliwatts per square centimeter (mW/cm^2). These values refer to the power of the ultrasound in a plane perpendicular to the axis of propagation of the beam. Since the power at any depth is not uniform over the entire plane, the *peak* intensity may be used (*spatial peak*) or the average (*spatial average*) may be used to express the power of a sound beam. Similarly, since imaging systems are pulsed, the *temporal average* or the *temporal peak intensity* may be used to describe a system.

The intensity output of a diagnostic imaging system is usually about 1 mW/cm^2. This is, however, the spatial average per temporal average output and is, therefore, the lowest possible figure. It is comparable to the power of continuous Doppler heart rate monitor systems. Because the spatial peak value may be 10 to 30 times the average for a focused beam, and since the pulse average may be 1000 times the temporal average, and finally because the temporal peak is 2 to 10 times the pulse average, the actual spatial peak–temporal peak intensity of an imaging system may be 20 to 300 W/cm^2. These are almost instantaneous spikes of energy. The impact on tissues of such pulsed power compared with the lower peak but similar average intensity of continuous Doppler systems is not known.

These considerations are of theoretical value in evaluating possible tissue effects of diagnostic imaging systems. The theoretical sources of tissue damage are heat production and cavitation. Cavitation refers to the generation and growth of tiny gas bubbles within molecular structures leading to potential physical or functional disruption.

The conclusion of the National Institutes of Health Consensus Development Conference on Obstetrical Ultrasound after careful study of all available documented evidence was that there is no evidence of ultrasonic damage to human conceptuses and that there is no good evidence of genetic damage. Some studies of single cell cultures exposed to ultrasound have shown a small increase in sister chromatid exchange rates, but there has been poor uniformity of method and there is great difficulty extrapolating such observations to the human system. Reduced litter weight in mice exposed to ultrasound during gestation has been reported and appears to be dose dependent, but exposure times and intensities relative to target mass are greatly exaggerated over the analogous situation of the human patient undergoing diagnostic sonography. Follow-up studies of infants exposed in utero to diagnostic ultrasound have not detected any adverse neonatal or later side effects from the fetal exposure. The safety of diagnostic ultrasound may never be completely settled, but at present there is no concrete evidence of human risk from diagnostic ultrasound.

Despite this apparent safety, it remains prudent to recommend the use of diagnostic ultrasound only when it might provide the answer to a clinically significant question. There are many appropriate clinical indications for sonographic evaluation of a pregnancy that we will consider. Casual uses of ultrasound cannot be promoted.

SUGGESTED READINGS

Baker ML, Dalrymple GV: Biological effects of diagnostic ultrasound: A review. *Radiology* 126:479–483, 1978.

Barnett SB, Kossoff G: Temporal peak intensity as a critical parameter in ultrasound dosimetry. *J Ultrasound Med* 3:385–389, 1984.

Brent RL: X-ray, microwave, and ultrasound—the real and unreal hazards. *Pediatr Ann* 9:12, 1980.

Carstensen EL, Gates AH: The effects of pulsed ultrasound on the fetus. *J Ultrasound Med* 3:145–147, 1984.

Goss SA: Sister chromatid exchange and ultrasound. *J Ultrasound Med* 3:463–470, 1984.

Kremkau F: Ultrasound instrumentation: Physical principles. In Callen PW (ed): *Ultrasonography in Obstetrics and Gynecology*. Philadelphia, WB Saunders, 1983, pp 313–324.

McDicken WN: *Diagnostic Ultrasonics: Principles and Use of Instruments*. New York, John Wiley & Sons, 1981

Stewart HC, Stewart HB, Moore RM, et al: Compilation of reported biological effects data and ultrasound exposure levels. *J Clin Ultrasound* 13:167–186, 1985.

Ziskin MC: Basic physics of ultrasound. In Saunders RC, James AE, Jr. (eds): *Ultrasonography in Obstetrics and Gynecology*. New York, Appleton-Century-Crofts, 1980, pp 1–14.

Chapter 2

Realtime Image Development

The use of the free-hand transducer of the realtime ultrasound machine to produce images of internal anatomy may be an unfamiliar or uncomfortable experience at first. The necessary elements of the rapid but orderly development of sonographic skills are time, practice, and discipline. Because the transducer is free hand, operators have the freedom to alter orientation in order to compose whatever image is desired. The technique requires the mental integration of multiple two-dimensional sonographic images into a three-dimensional anatomical aggregate. The interpretation of serial anatomical tomograms is a common experience in medicine. Operators must use their knowledge of anatomy not only to interpret images but also to guide the movement of the transducer in composing images of the desired structures.

None of these requirements is difficult. The mental/manual skills are quickly developed with practice. The transducer becomes an extension of an operator's mind in the composition of anatomical images of the fetus.

The most common mistakes made by sonographers early in their experience with ultrasound are excessively rapid movement of the transducer, incomplete examinations, and avoiding anatomy they do not understand. Each tomographic image produced by the scanner is full of detail. It is a common mistake to move the transducer too fast to appreciate the information available. At first, it is wiser to make painfully deliberate moves, studying each picture carefully and deciding exactly where to move next. The time invested at this point will pay dividends later. Speed will come with time and experience, but only if time is taken early to lay the foundation of deliberate, well-organized habits.

FORMAT

There is no law that requires a consistent orientation of the display screen to maternal anatomy. It is just prudent for sonographers to try to minimize the number of spatial variables they have to deal with in sorting out anatomy. Experienced sonographers maintain a consistent relationship between the orientation of the display screen and the position of the patient. When the transducer is transverse on the patient's abdomen, the right side of the display screen should show the left side of the patient (Fig 2-1). It is as if one is at the foot of the bed looking at the patient. This is analogous to the proper orientation of a radiograph when viewed. When the transducer is longitudinal on the patient, the orientation should have the maternal diaphragm or uterine fundus to the left, and the maternal pelvis to the right, as if the operator were to the right of the bed observing the patient (Fig 2-2). These conventions might seem awkward at first, but a little time spent with them now will pay off later in time saved and confusion avoided.

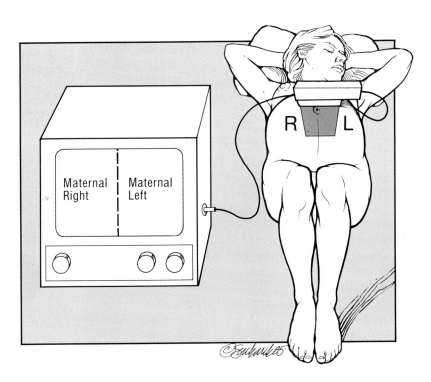

Fig 2-1. Transverse format. When scanning the maternal abdomen in the transverse plane the display screen should be oriented to maintain the maternal left side to the right of the screen and the maternal right side to the left of the screen.

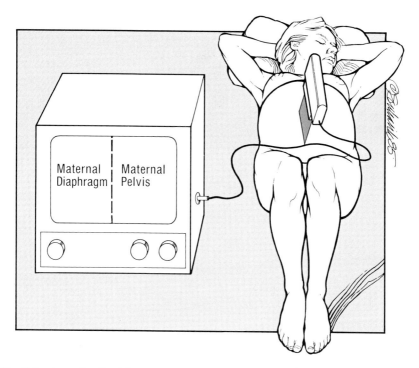

| Maternal Diaphragm | Maternal Pelvis |

Fig 2-2. Longitudinal format. When scanning the maternal abdomen in a longitudinal plane the recommended format maintains maternal pelvis to the right of the display screen and maternal diaphragm or uterine fundus to the left.

THE MOVES

There are three basic movements possible with the linear array transducer, and there are analogous moves appropriate for the sector scanner. The first is a sliding movement that does not change the angle of entry of the scan plane or the relation of the transducer to the long axis of the mother (Fig 2-3). This movement might be individually useful for finding the correct cranial level for a biparietal diameter once other conditions have been satisfied. The second type of movement is a rotational change of the relationship of the long axis of the transducer to that of the mother (Fig 2-4). Such a move might individually be used to capture the entire length of the femur or any other long bone once a smaller portion of it is seen.

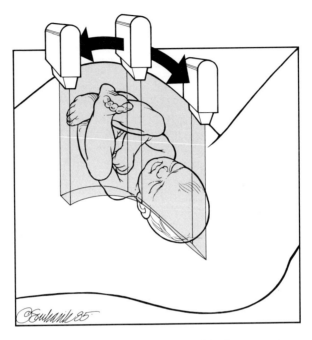

Fig 2-3. Sliding motion. A sliding motion with the transducer produces a three-dimensional field of view (shaded area).

Finally, the angle of entry may be separately altered without moving the transducer contact point at all (Fig 2-5). In combination with the other moves, this is often necessary in achieving an ideal angle for a variety of images and measurements, including biparietal diameter and abdominal circumference. In practice, few operators use these moves alone but instead use them together in complex combinations. However, at first, it is useful to practice each individually, to appreciate how they might be used to develop a desired image from an imperfect one.

THE START

An organized, methodical ultrasound examination helps ensure that each scan will be done completely and properly (Table 2-1). Each operator should construct or adopt a definite checklist of information and anatomy to be included in each examination. It is useful to begin with a general survey of uterine contents and adnexae, in both longitudinal and transverse planes

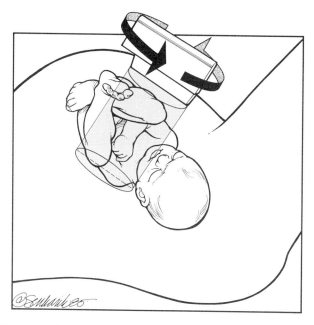

Fig 2-4. Rotational movement. A pure rotational movement produces a field of view in the shape of a cylinder (shaded area).

relative to the mother. The operator begins by placing the transducer in the suprapubic midline longitudinally. The transducer is slowly angled from side to side and is slid cranially until the limit of the uterus is reached and then moved just beyond the limit of the uterus. With this type of survey the sonographer should be able to identify the number of fetuses and the presentation, to begin to assess placental location, to assess fetal viability through the identification of heart movement, and to judge the relative volume of amniotic fluid. The operator then replaces the transducer transversely in the lower midline and again slides it slowly cranially, confirming or completing the above observations. Proceeding beyond the margins of the uterus allows the detection of significant adnexal pathologic conditions such as ovarian cysts. Once the position of the fetus is determined, necessary measurements of fetal dimensions can be made. These will be discussed in detail in later chapters. After the desired fetal dimensions are recorded, a careful survey of fetal anatomy should be performed to search for sonographically visible malformations. Orientation of the transducer should be adapted to the fetus once the general survey of the uterus is completed in order to produce recognizable anatomy more easily. It is poor

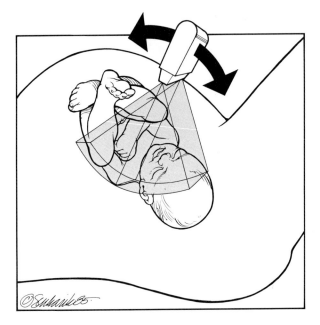

Fig 2-5. Angle movement. Changing only the angle of entry at the skin surface produces a total field of view (shaded area).

Table 2-1. Outline of an Ultrasound Examination

Uterine Survey—Longitudinal/Transverse
• Fetal number
• Fetal position
• Fetal viability
• Placental location and texture
• Amniotic fluid volume
Fetal Dimensions
• Biparietal diameter
• Femur or humerus length
• Mean abdominal diameter or circumference
• Mean head diameter or circumference
Fetal Anatomy
• Craniospinal
• Thoracic
• Abdominal
• Urinary tract
• Long bones

practice to attempt to interpret oblique fetal anatomy from carelessly composed images. Every attempt should be made, therefore, to produce deliberate transverse and longitudinal fetal images, avoiding off-axis cuts.

THE IMAGES

Both the skill necessary to develop clear and appropriate images of fetal anatomy and the visual ability to discriminate the anatomy represented are developed as a result of time, patience, and practice. In the beginning it will help to focus on easily recognized fetal structures such as the skull, the heart, or the spine. Sonographers must use their knowledge of gross anatomy to develop deliberate images of adjacent fetal organs. Slow, methodical movements of the transducer are used. A survey of the major fetal organ systems is listed in Table 2-1. A complete ultrasound examination for the beginning sonographer might require up to an hour, but with experience and practice this can be reduced to 15 minutes.

Chapter 3

Normal Fetal Sonographic Anatomy

As early as 5 weeks post menstruation a gestational sac may be seen within the uterus using realtime ultrasound. By 8 weeks' gestation a vague fetal outline may be seen and heart action should be apparent. By 12 weeks' gestation the fetus has form and individual limbs may be imaged and measured. If a definite cranium is not seen after 14 weeks, anencephaly must be suspected. This orderly progression of sonographic visibility of fetal anatomy using ultrasound is continued throughout pregnancy. At each successive stage of pregnancy greater detail is possible in the visualization of fetal structures. We will study the normal fetus by regions. In many cases gestational age is not precisely relevant, but when it is, the specific impact of gestational age on anatomical appearance will be mentioned.

CRANIOSPINAL ANATOMY

The fetal cranium should be seen with good quality realtime equipment by 14 weeks' gestation, often even earlier. From 14 to 17 weeks' gestation, when studied in the standard occipitofrontal plane used to measure a biparietal diameter, the cranium assumes a typical oval or egg shape. Visually, the dominant intracranial organ is the echogenic choroid plexus (Fig 3-1). At a slightly more caudal level, the frontal horns of the lateral ventricle may be seen and measured on either side of the anterior midline (Fig 3-2). The lateral margins of the lateral ventricles are most clearly seen when the midline is exactly perpendicular to the direction of the sound beam. Prior to 17 weeks' gestation the ratio of the width of either anterior horn to the hemispheric width (midline to inner skull table at the widest point) in the same plane does not normally exceed 0.50. Hydrocephalus may be suspected if this ratio appears larger than this limit. Beyond 17 weeks' gestation, owing to the growth of the skull and brain but not proportionate growth of the ventricles, the ventriculohemispheric (V/H) ratio decreases

29

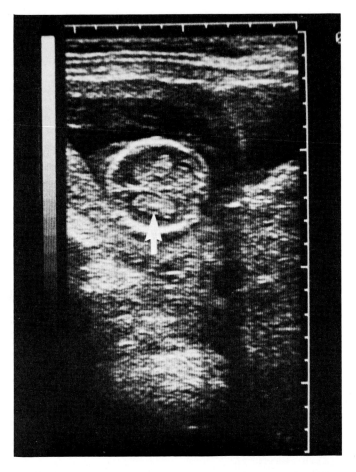

Fig 3-1. Choroid plexus. In this occipitofrontal scan plane just above the thalami of the fetal cranium at approximately 16 weeks' gestational age, the choroid plexus (arrow) is seen as an echogenic soft tissue structure located within each hemisphere.

and falls below 0.33. The actual width of the anterior horns rarely exceeds 9 mm prior to 22 weeks and 11 mm from 22 to 32 weeks and should remain less than 12 mm beyond that time.

From 20 weeks' gestation to term more detailed intracranial anatomy is seen, including the cerebellar hemispheres within the posterior fossa just posterior to the brain stem (Fig 3-3). The thalami of the midbrain are just

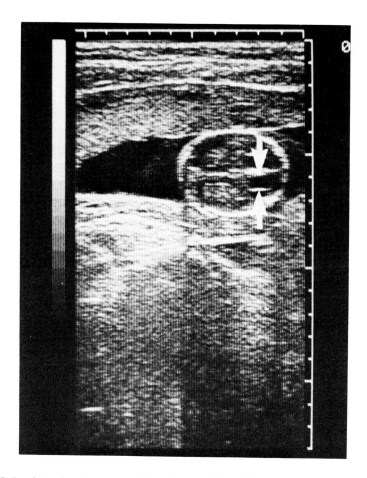

Fig 3-2. Anterior horns of lateral ventricles. This is an occipitofrontal scan of the 17-week fetal cranium caudal to that in Figure 3-1 demonstrating the anterior horns of the lateral ventricles. The two arrows bracket the measurement of a frontal horn.

behind the cavum septum pellucidum (Fig 3-4). The third ventricle located in the midline between the thalami and the fourth ventricle between the cerebellar hemispheres in the posterior fossa are both normally not seen unless they are dilated as the result of a pathologic condition.

The fetal spine should be examined both longitudinally and transversely to provide the maximum sensitivity in diagnosing abnormalities. When seen transversely, the neural canal may be seen to be contained within three bony

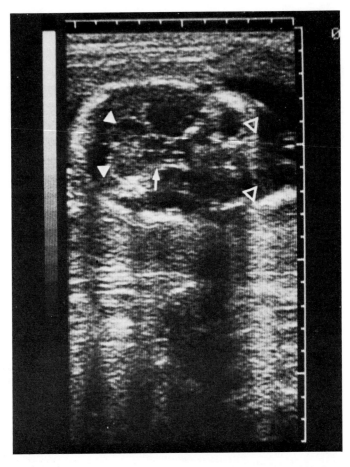

Fig 3-3. Posterior fossa. This view of the fetal cranium is slightly more caudal in level than that in Figure 3-2 and illustrates the posterior fossa with cerebellar hemispheres (solid triangles), the brain stem (arrow), and the orbits (open triangles).

or echogenic centers (Fig 3-5*A*). Two are posterior (dorsal) and slightly paramedian, and a single midline center is just anterior to the others. These represent the centers for the vertebral body and the neural arches and appear on early scan as the points of an equilateral triangle. Transverse scanning should be performed serially from cranium to sacrum, with careful attention to the relationships of these points to each other, particularly the posterolateral points. Spinal defects typically result in lateral displacement of the

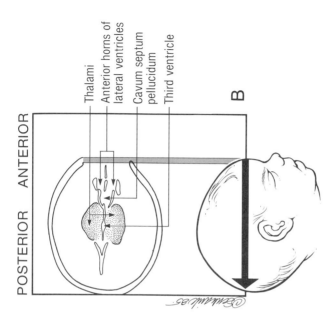

POSTERIOR ANTERIOR

Thalami
Anterior horns of lateral ventricles
Cavum septum pellucidum
Third ventricle

B

Fig 3-4. Thalami: (*A*) This occipitofrontal sonogram of a fetal cranium at the level of the thalami (t), cavum septum pellucidum, and frontal horns of lateral ventricles is approximately the correct level for a measurement of a biparietal diameter. (*B*) Diagram emphasizes the important anatomical elements visible on the scan.

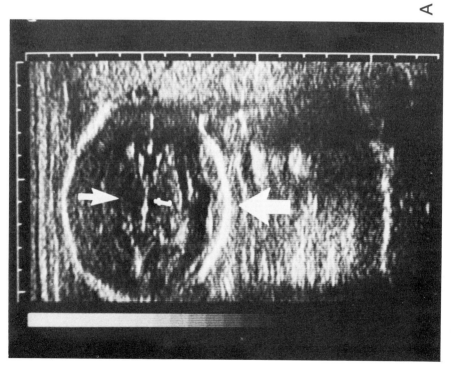

A

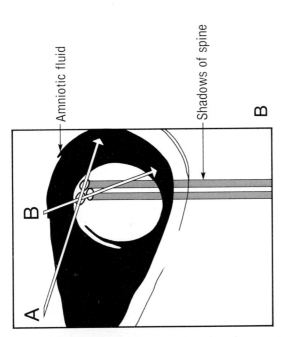

Amniotic fluid

Shadows of spine

Fig 3-5. (A) Transverse spine. This transverse scan of the fetal abdomen at approximately 15 weeks' gestation shows the spinal elements as three bright echogenic centers in the posterior aspect of the fetus. Normally, these centers appear as the points of a triangle. (B) Transverse spine with proper longitudinal scan planes. This sketch of the accompanying sonogram illustrates two possible planes for longitudinal scanning. Longitudinal views of the fetal spine from each of these two possible view points are illustrated in Figure 3-6.

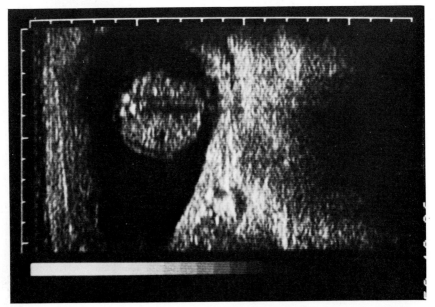

lateral posterior elements and a flattening of the normal triangular arrangement, and the posterior centers grow closer to the fetal skin surface.

A longitudinal scan of the normal fetal spine shows two parallel rows of echogenic spinal elements. Such an image can capture only two of the three rows of spinal echocenters in any one scan plane (Fig 3-5*B*). The most sensitive longitudinal scan for the diagnosis of spina bifida is of the posterolateral spinal echocenters since it is these that are most significantly displaced with spina bifida (Fig 3-6).

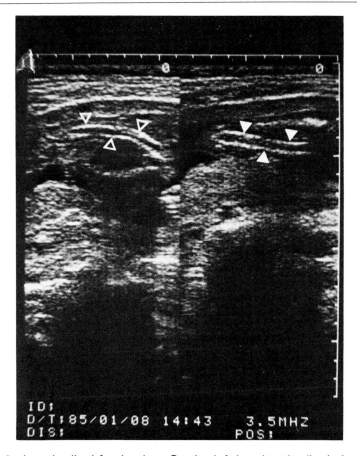

Fig 3-6. Longitudinal fetal spine. On the left is a longitudinal view of a fetal spine (open triangles) obtained when the scan plane is oriented similar to plane B as illustrated in Figure 3-5*B*. The view on the right side of this figure is a longitudinal scan of a fetal spine (solid triangles) obtained when the transducer is oriented as illustrated by plane A in Figure 3-5*B*.

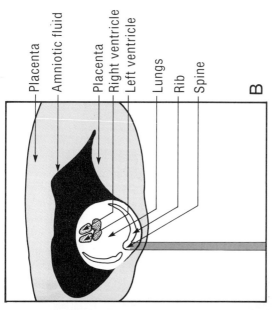

Placenta
Amniotic fluid
Placenta
Right ventricle
Left ventricle
Lungs
Rib
Spine

B

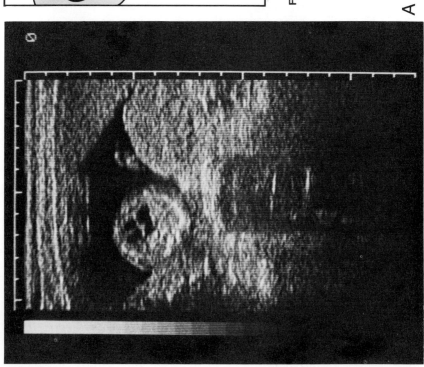

A

Fig 3-7. Transverse fetal chest. (*A*) Transverse scan of the mid chest of a 17-week fetus illustrating the four chambers and lung fields. (*B*) Diagram of major anatomical features shown on the sonogram.

CHEST ANATOMY

The fetal chest contains the lungs, heart, and great vessels. All of these structures may be evaluated. The normal fetal heart occupies the central chest and with transverse scanning is shown to comprise four chambers: two ventricles and two atria (Fig 3-7). The best plane for cardiac imaging is one that is slightly oblique, parallel to the fetal ribs aligned with an intercostal space. The long axis of the fetal heart is seen inclined slightly to the fetal left side. The mean cardiac diameter (average of a long and a short axis measurement) is usually less than 55% of the average chest diameter in the same four-chamber view plane. The ventricles should demonstrate synchronous contractile activity on realtime viewing, and the ventricles are of roughly equal diameter at their base. The left ventricle is the more posterior of the two, and its cavity is relatively free of internal echos. The apex of the left ventricle is typically more sharply defined, and the left ventricle may appear slightly longer than the right. The right ventricle is the more anterior of the two, with noticeably more apical irregularity. Commonly a prominent papillary muscle is seen crossing the cavity of the right ventricle to a leaflet of the tricuspid valve (Fig 3-8). The atria are thin walled and roughly of equal size. M-mode (motion mode) fetal echocardiography may be useful to study cardiac rhythm and to discriminate arrhythmias of the ventricles or atria.

The lungs fill the chest on either side of the heart and present a diffusely echogenic appearance. It is abnormal to see any discrete cystic cavity within the chest alongside the heart. It is also abnormal to see the lungs outlined by fluid within the pleural space. In examining the chest apart from the cardiac chambers, it is very important to be sure the scan planes are perpendicular to the spine. Oblique views might include a part of the stomach with the lower left ventricle of the heart and produce the false appearance of a cystic structure within the chest that might be mistakenly interpreted as herniated stomach. In addition to heart and lungs it is possible to visualize the aorta and the aortic arch within the chest (Fig 3-9), and with some patience and effort, the aortic and pulmonary valves may be seen.

ABDOMINAL ANATOMY

The fetal abdomen should be scanned both longitudinally and transversely (Fig 3-10). Transverse abdominal scans, in addition to showing spinal anatomy, will show the fetal stomach in the left upper abdomen (Fig 3-11) and the fetal kidneys as circular soft tissue organs on either side of the spine in the posterior mid abdomen. The umbilicus should appear as a discrete,

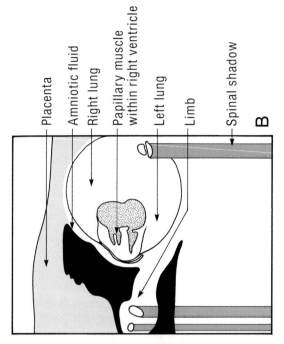

Placenta

Amniotic fluid

Right lung

Papillary muscle
within right ventricle

Left lung

Limb

Spinal shadow

B

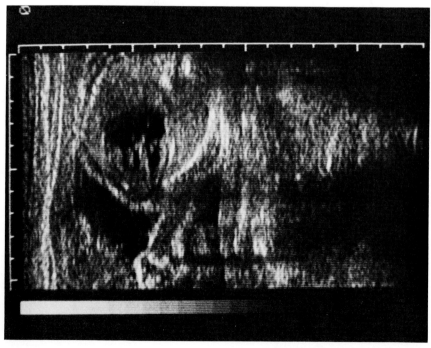

A

Fig 3-8. Normal cardiac anatomy. (*A*) Transverse sonogram of a fetal chest at approximately 26 weeks' gestation. (*B*) Diagram of the major anatomical features shown on the sonogram.

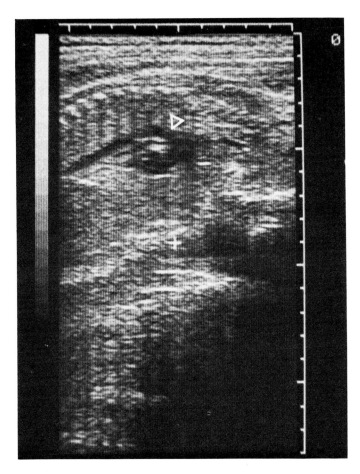

Fig 3-9. Aortic arch. Longitudinal scan of the fetal chest demonstrating the aortic arch. The aortic arch is echolucent (black) owing to the liquid blood within it. The open triangle indicates a mid aortic arch within the fetal chest.

abrupt, entry of umbilical vessels through the lower anterior midline abdominal wall (Fig 3-12), and the fetal bladder should be found in the anterior midline of the fetal pelvis (Fig 3-13) and with care is virtually always seen by 18 weeks' gestation. The general contour of the fetal abdomen is circular, but since it is soft and pliable, considerable distortion is possible, particularly with oligohydramnios.

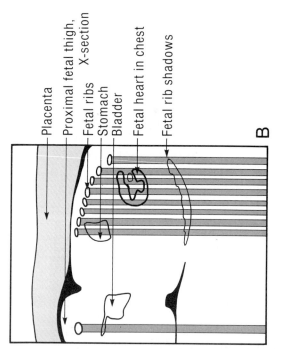

Placenta

Proximal fetal thigh,
X-section

Fetal ribs

Stomach

Bladder

Fetal heart in chest

Fetal rib shadows

B

Fig 3-10. Fetal trunk. (*A*) Longitudinal scan of the fetal trunk at approximately 20 weeks' gestation. The scan plane enters the fetus at approximately the midaxillary line. (*B*) Diagram of the sonogram highlighting major anatomical features.

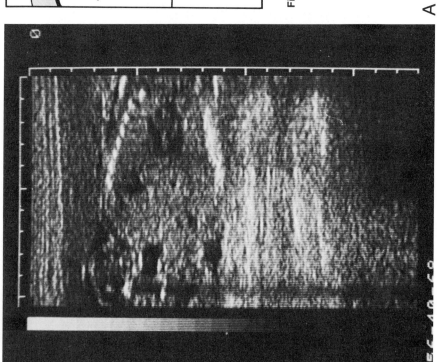

A

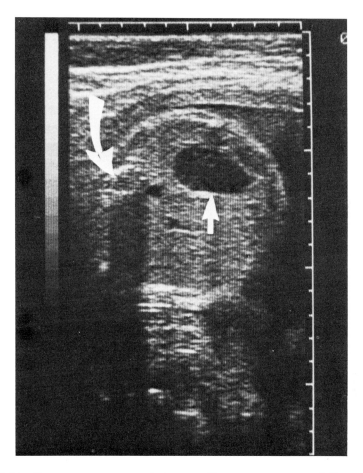

Fig 3-11. Transverse upper abdomen. Transverse scan of the upper
fetal abdomen demonstrating the fetal spine (curved arrow)
with appropriate spinal shadow and fetal stomach (straight
arrow) in a normal fetus.

Prior to about 24 weeks' gestation, the kidneys are not normally well
outlined. They are seen on transverse fetal scan only as areas of lower
echodensity on either side of the spine in the mid abdomen (Fig 3-14).
However, later in gestation, the kidneys become well outlined sonographically by perirenal fat deposition, which results in bright echos and clearly
outlined kidneys (Fig 3-15). The kidneys may be studied longitudinally, as

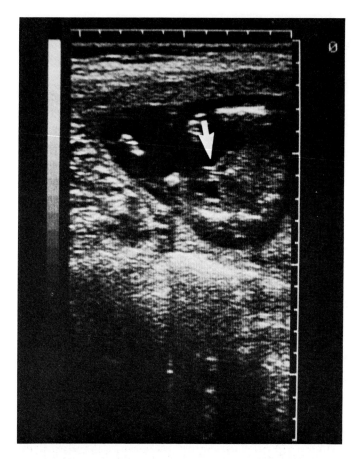

Fig 3-12. Umbilicus. This transverse scan of the lower abdomen of a fetus demonstrates a normal insertion of an umbilical cord (straight arrow). Normally the cord inserts in the abdominal wall abruptly, and there is good angulation here.

---

well as transversely (Fig 3-16), and the renal papillae often appear quite echolucent (dark). Normal growth charts have been reported for both longitudinal and transverse dimensions of the kidneys, and these norms may be useful for the diagnosis of disease. The ratio of the kidney circumference to the abdominal circumference at the same level remains close to 0.30 throughout pregnancy.

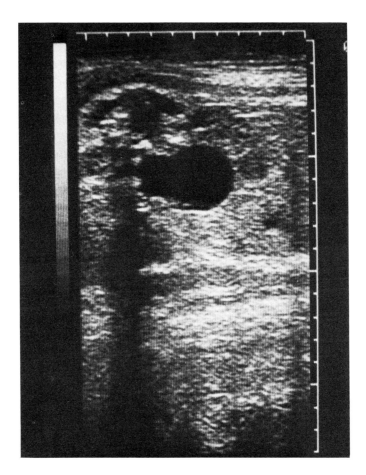

Fig 3-13. Normal bladder. The fetal bladder is an echolucent (black) structure in the anterior mid pelvis.

SKELETAL ANATOMY

The proximal and distal long bones of all limbs may be imaged and measured with contemporary realtime equipment (Fig 3-17). Side to side symmetry of long bone dimensions should be nearly perfect. The observation of any irregularities of shape should be carefully recorded.

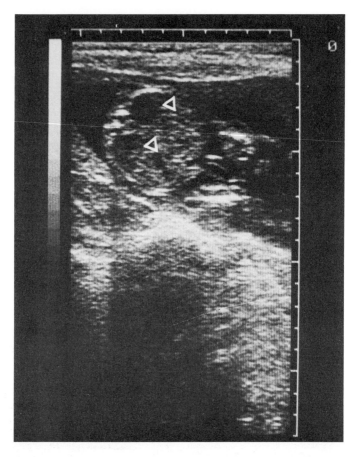

Fig 3-14. Early fetal kidneys. Prior to 24 weeks' gestation, fetal kidneys are seen only as circular echolucent areas in the posterior mid abdomen on the transverse scan (open triangles).

CONCLUSION

The student of sonography is strongly urged to explore and examine each of these areas of fetal anatomy methodically with each examination. Considerable confidence will be developed with time and practice, and the occasional abnormal case will be more easily and reliably identified.

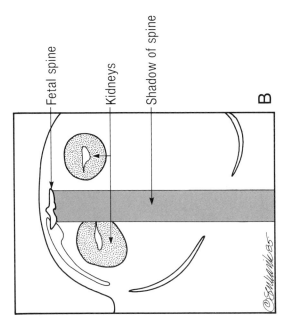

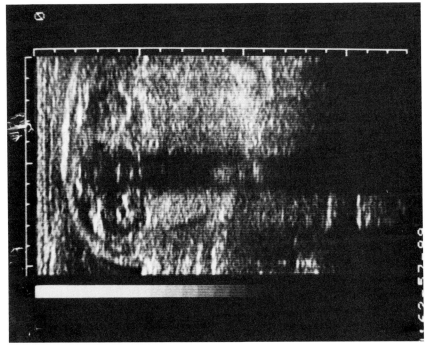

Fig 3-15. Late fetal kidneys. (A) Later in gestation, the kidneys are sharply outlined by perinephric fat. (B) Diagram of the sonogram illustrates major points of anatomy.

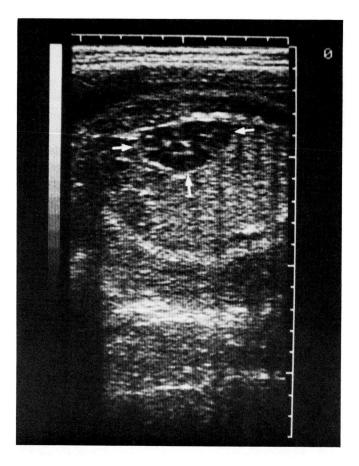

Fig 3-16. Longitudinal kidney. This longitudinal view of the fetal kidney (within arrows) illustrates the occasional striking echolucent appearance of the normal fetal kidney.

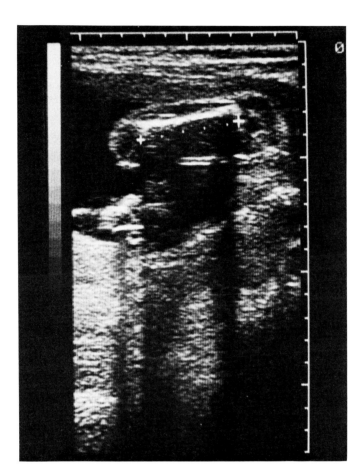

Fig 3-17. Fetal long bones. This longitudinal view of the fetal femur illustrates a typical appearance of fetal long bones. Note the striking shadow, which may be used to assist in identifying the true extent of a fetal bone.

SUGGESTED READINGS

Allan LD, Tynan MJ, Campbell S, et al: Echocardiographic and anatomical correlates in the fetus. *Br Heart J* 44:444-451, 1980.

Allan LD, Tynan M, Campbell S, et al: Normal fetal cardiac anatomy—a basis for the echocardiographic detection of abnormalities. *Prenatal Diagnosis* 1:131-139, 1981.

Bertagnoli L, Lalatta F, Gallicchio R: Quantitative characterization of the growth of the fetal kidney. *J Clin Ultrasound* 11:349-356, 1983.

Bowie JD, Rosenberg ER, Andreatte RF, et al: The changing sonographic appearance of fetal kidneys during pregnancy. *J Ultrasound Med* 2:505–507, 1983.

Brandt TD, Neiman HL, Dragowski MJ: Ultrasound assessment of normal renal dimensions. *J Ultrasound Med* 1:49–52, 1982.

Filly RA, Callen PW: Ultrasonographic evaluation of normal fetal anatomy. In Saunders RC, James AE, Jr. (eds): *Ultrasonography in Obstetrics and Gynecology.* New York, Appleton-Century-Crofts, 1980, pp 91–110.

Fiske CE, Filly RA: Ultrasound evaluation of the normal and abnormal fetal neural axis. *Radiol Clin North Am* 20:285–296, 1983.

Grannum P, Bracken M, Silverman R, Hobbins JC: Assessment of fetal kidney size in normal gestations by comparison of ratio of kidney circumference to abdominal circumference. *Am J Obstet Gynecol* 136:249–254, 1980.

Grant EG, Schellinger D, Richardson JD: Realtime ultrasonography of the posterior fossa. *J Ultrasound Med* 2:73–87, 1983.

Jeanty P, Romero R, Cantraine F, et al: Fetal cardiac dimensions—a potential tool for the diagnosis of congenital heart defects. *J Ultrasound Med* 3:359–364, 1984.

Yamaguchi DT, Lee FYL: Ultrasonic evaluation of the fetal heart. *Am J Obstet Gynecol* 134:422–430, 1979.

Chapter 4

Sonographic Gestational Age Assignment

The length of a normal pregnancy is 280 days from the first day of the last normal menstrual period in the case of regular 28-day cycles. Based on clinical criteria, including last menstrual period and a compatible early physical examination, onset of labor may be predicted within 3 weeks in 90% of cases. Irregular menstrual cycles or historical inaccuracies account for many of the observed discrepancies between actual and estimated dates of confinement.

An accurate alternative to clinical assignment of gestational age is necessary when the menstrual history is unclear, or altered by recent medications or pregnancy, and in the case of the high-risk pregnancy for which accurate gestational age assignment is a high clinical priority.

Assignment of gestational age using sonographic fetal dimensions is based on the empirical relationship between a variety of fetal dimensions and gestational age. Although the observed correlation is fairly precise, there is a natural variability at any point of any such relationship. It is of practical importance to remember that with few exceptions, all reference populations used as the basis for fetal sonographic dimensional growth charts have been clinically dated. Furthermore, since in any clinically dated population there is a variation of $+/-$ 2 weeks in the achievement of important developmental milestones such as lung maturity or the onset of labor, it is inappropriate to assume that sonographic dating can predict any of these milestones better than accurate clinical dates. Also, any measurement method will involve a degree of technical variability that ought to be added to the biological variability of the reference population. Finally, fetal growth may be altered within any reference group, possibly as a result of high altitude, ethnic, and/or socioeconomic factors. Such factors could affect the validity of certain data for use in estimating gestational age in a patient who is not subject to similar altitude or social influences.

The evolution of sonographic techniques for gestational dating has seen gradual standardization of method and steady improvement in technical precision.[1-5] Early inconsistency in the assumed speed of sound in soft tissue has been settled, and the accepted average speed of sound is set at 1540 meters per second. Scan planes and measurement landmarks have become more uniform. Repeated analysis of single and combined multiple indices of fetal size has resulted in improved clinical precision.

We will examine multiple sonographic parameters of gestational age. All are more accurate estimators of gestational age (EGA) before 20 weeks' gestation than they are later in pregnancy. None can be expected to predict clinical events more accurately than an accurate last menstrual period. Ultrasonic gestational age assignment compares a selected fetal dimension from a pregnancy in need of gestational age confirmation with the regression mean for that dimension calculated from a carefully dated reference population. The reported statistical variability refers only to the variability of the specific dimension at the indicated gestational age. This variability is not truly a measure of predictive accuracy.

Given equal technical proficiency, the result from the earliest of any series of sonographic assessments is the best estimate of gestational age. Subsequent examinations will reflect the quality of interval growth, not improved accuracy of EGA. A due date must not be serially revised because serial ultrasound evaluations provide conflicting data. It is equally inappropriate to revise the estimated due date on the basis of ultrasound data if the clinical gestational age is within the statistical range of variability of the sonographic EGA. It is generally not recommended after 20 weeks' gestation to revise a gestational age for a discrepancy of less than 2 weeks.

METHODOLOGY

Biparietal Diameter

The fetal cranium was one of the first fetal structures reliably visualized with ultrasound. The biparietal diameter (BPD) of the fetal cranium was chosen as an early index of growth because of this reliable visibility. The BPD is the largest diameter of the cranium perpendicular to the midline in an occipitofrontal scan plane.

There are many published reports relating BPD to gestational age. No two of these studies are precisely identical in results or design. EGA varies from one chart to another for the same BPD measurement by as much as 2 weeks. In an effort to standardize the method, composite BPD growth curves have been derived from the data of multiple comparable individual studies.[5,6] These composite BPD charts appear to be more appropriate for the individual practitioner because averaging minimizes a variety of potential technical biases between institutions and investigators. A composite BPD growth chart is provided in Table 4-1.[5,7,8]

The correct level of the fetal cranium for the measurement of the BPD is achieved when the scan plane is perpendicular to the midline of the fetal skull in an occipitofrontal orientation just above the orbits. This is the largest plane of the fetal head and provides an oval skull outline with a centered midline and symmetrical parietal bone curvature.

The easiest approach to develop such an image is to align the transducer with the fetal spine, slide the transducer cranially until the head is seen, and then turn it 90°. An inappropriate coronal scan plane will produce a more circular outline of the fetal cranium if it is a dorsal coronal view (Fig 4-1) or will demonstrate fetal orbits if it is a ventral coronal view (Fig 4-2). Once the appropriate oval cranial shape is seen, the angle of the scan plane should be adjusted to center the midline (Fig 4-3). The transducer is then moved up or down to produce the largest oval cranial outline. If intracranial anatomy is visible, the cavum septum pellucidum and the thalami are usually seen (see Fig 3-4). The correct BPD is the largest transcranial diameter perpendicular to the midline in this plane. The measurement is made from the leading edge (closest to transducer) of the proximal skull table to the leading edge of the distal table (Fig 4-4). With BPD, as with other dating dimensions, several independent determinations should be done until the results are consistent within 1 mm. The EGA may be estimated from this BPD by referring to Table 4-1.

BPD may be measured from 14 to 42 weeks' gestation. The accuracy, however, decreases as pregnancy progresses (see Table 4-1). Clearly, earlier is better. Furthermore, there are certain clinical situations such as persistent breech or severe oligohydramnios in which the BPD is particularly inaccurate owing to physical distortion or even totally unavailable.[9,10] When the vertex is deeply engaged in the pelvis, a correct plane from which to measure BPD may not be accessible. Distortion of cranial shape renders the BPD inaccurate as an index of gestational age. The examiner must be prepared to evaluate cranial shape, as well as be ready to use some alternate dimension to BPD as the situation requires.

The *cephalic index* (CI) is an assessment of skull shape that is calculated by dividing the largest transverse cranial diameter by the occipitofrontal diameter. The normal ratio is about 0.78. When calculating the CI, the transverse and longitudinal diameters should be measured in a similar way in the same scan plane, from outer edge of skull table to outer edge of the opposite skull table. This allows these same diameters to be used to calculate head circumference. A CI below 0.73 (dolichocephaly) or above 0.83

Table 4-1. Fetal Growth Parameters (mm)

Gestational Age	Biparietal Diameter[5]	Femur Length[7]	Humerus Length[7]	Head Circumference[8]	Average Head Diameter	Abdominal Circumference[8]	Average Abdominal Diameter
14	28	15	15	101	32	84	27
15	32	18	18	114	36	95	30
16	36	20	21	128	41	106	34
17	39	23	23	141	45	117	37
18	42	26	26	154	49	128	41
19	45	29	28	167	53	139	44
20	48	32	31	179	57	150	48
21	51	35	33	192	61	161	51
22	54	37	35	204	65	172	55
23	58	40	37	215	68	183	58
24	61	42	39	227	72	194	62
25	64	45	41	238	76	205	65
26	67	48	44	249	79	216	69
27	70	50	46	259	82	227	72
28	72	53	48	269	86	238	76
29	75	55	49	279	89	249	79
30	78	57	51	288	92	260	83
31	80	60	53	297	95	271	86
32	82	62	55	306	97	282	90
33	85	64	57	314	100	293	93
34	87	67	59	322	102	304	97
35	88	69	60	329	105	315	100
36	90	71	62	336	107	326	104
37	92	73	64	342	109	337	107
38	93	76	66	348	111	348	111
39	94	78	67	354	113	359	114
40	95	80	69	359	114	370	118

95% Confidence Intervals

Biparietal Diameter — 14–20 weeks ± 7 days / 20–30 weeks ± 10 days / 30–40 weeks ± 21 days

Femur or Humerus Length — 14–20 weeks ± 7 days / 20–30 weeks ± 10 days / 30–40 weeks ± 12 days

Head Circumference (Diameter) — 14–28 weeks ± 1.5 cm / 28–40 weeks ± 2.5 cm

Abdominal Circumference (Diameter) — 14–40 weeks ± 13%

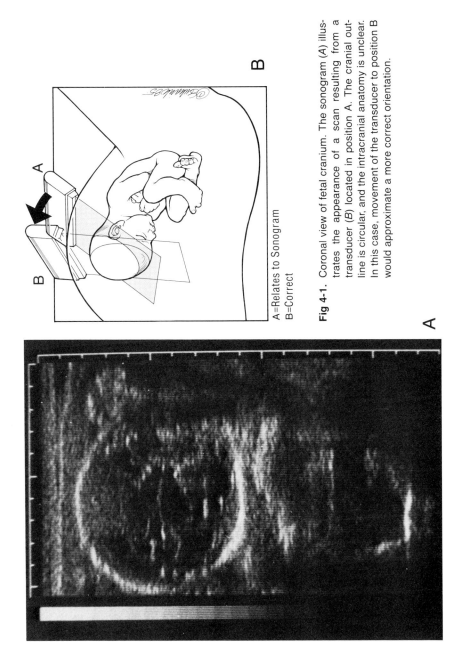

A=Relates to Sonogram
B=Correct

Fig 4-1. Coronal view of fetal cranium. The sonogram (A) illustrates the appearance of a scan resulting from a transducer (B) located in position A. The cranial outline is circular, and the intracranial anatomy is unclear. In this case, movement of the transducer to position B would approximate a more correct orientation.

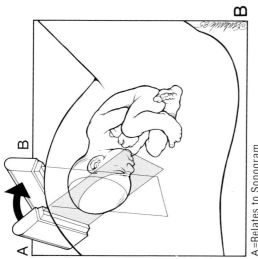

A=Relates to Sonogram
B=Correct

Fig 4-2. Anterior coronal view. The sonogram (A) illustrates the image produced by the transducer (B) located in position A. In this case the intracranial anatomy is obscure, the cranial outline is circular, and the orbits (arrows) are seen. Movement of the transducer toward position B should result in a more correct orientation.

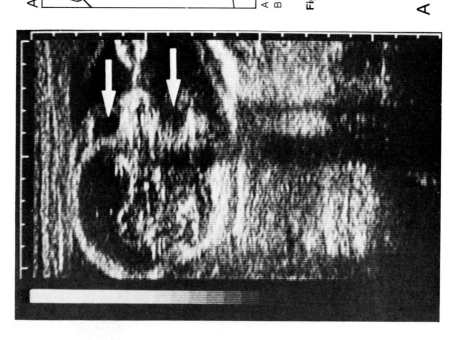

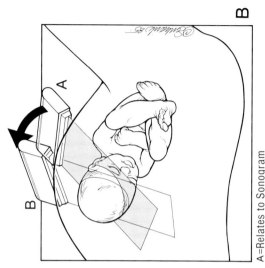

A=Relates to Sonogram
B=Correct

Fig 4-3. Off-axis cranial view. The sonogram (A) illustrates the visual appearance of a scan produced when the transducer (B) is in position A. Intracranial anatomy is unclear, and parietal echos are asymmetrical. In this case the transducer should be moved toward position B to normalize the scan plane.

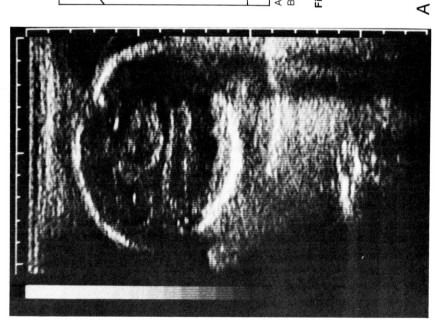

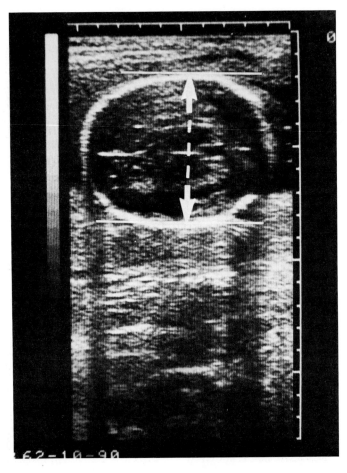

Fig 4-4. Biparietal diameter. As the result of the movements described in Figures 4-1 through 4-3, an appropriate occipitofrontal scan plane perpendicular to the midline should result. The largest diameter of this cranium perpendicular to the midline from leading edge to leading edge constitutes the biparietal diameter.

(brachycephaly) indicates distortion and that the measured BPD is not representative of the gestational age of that fetus. The brachycephalic head has a short occipitofrontal axis and a broad BPD. The average of the two diameters measured from outer edge to outer edge multiplied by 3.1416 gives an accurate estimate of head circumference (Fig 4-5). Head circumference may also be directly estimated by either mechanical or electronic

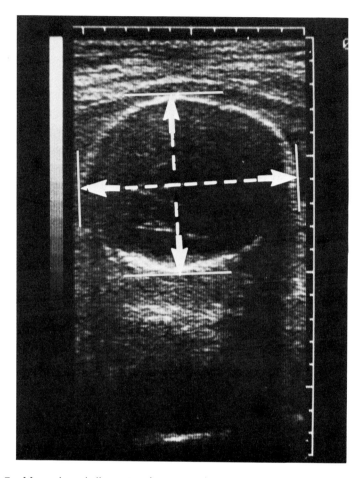

Fig 4-5. Mean head diameter. In approximately the same scan plane as Figure 4-4, two diameters are measured from outer edge to outer edge both transversely and longitudinally. The average of these two diameters then constitutes the mean head diameter.

perimeter measurement techniques (Fig 4-6). There is little difference between head circumference calculated from mean head diameter and that derived from perimeter measurement. Head circumference from perimeter techniques is often slightly augmented by minor errors of the operator in following the margin of the cranium. The use of head circumference primarily to date a fetus prevents head distortion from altering the EGA and is

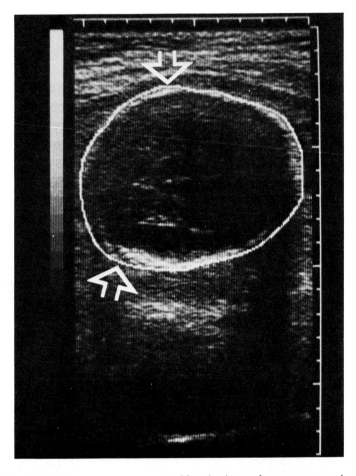

Fig 4-6. Perimeter measurement. Head circumference may be estimated from either mean head diameter or by perimeter measurement. Electronic perimeter measurement involves a risk of error owing to failure to follow the skull edge (arrows) properly.

---

recommended by many authorities over BPD as a dating parameter. Table 4-1 includes both head circumference and mean head diameter.

Femur and Humerus Length

Measurement of the fetal femur or humerus length has become popular as realtime equipment capable of easily imaging these mobile fetal limbs has become available.[7,11,12]

Here again, there are multiple growth charts relating long bone dimensions to gestational age, and again none of them are precisely identical.[7,11-14] The biological variability of the femur measurements of a reference population increases with gestational age, and the earlier in pregnancy the femur is measured, the more precise the estimate of gestational age is seen to be. Femur-based EGA before 20 weeks' gestation is comparably accurate to BPD (see Table 4-1).[11,14]

Passive physical distortion of the long bones related to either presentation or oligohydramnios is rare, and inability to image the femur or humerus is

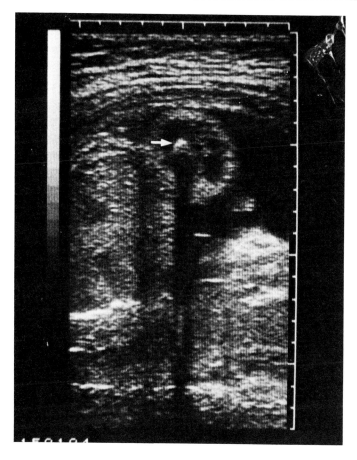

Fig 4-7. Transverse thigh. The transverse scan of the fetal thigh illustrates the appearance of the femur in cross section (arrow). Rotation of the transducer should gradually reveal greater portions of the femur.

equally rare. Therefore, in any situation in which the BPD appears distorted or is unavailable, femur and humerus both represent logical, equal alternatives. In the third trimester femur length appears to be a more accurate estimator of gestational age than BPD.[7,11,14] This superiority may be important if gestational age must unavoidably be evaluated late in pregnancy.

Technique

Imaging the femur may be accomplished by aligning the transducer with the spine, sliding it to the caudal end of the fetus, and rotating the transducer slowly toward the ventral aspect of the fetus until the femur comes into view. Alternatively, the transducer may be placed transverse to the fetal spine and moved caudally until a portion of one femur is seen transversely, within the usually flexed thigh (Fig 4-7). Often only a fraction of a femur will be seen at first, and rotation of the transducer is necessary to capture a greater length of the bone (Fig 4-8). Rotation and slight angling will convince the operator that the entire length has been captured. The image must then be frozen and the length from end to end parallel to the shaft measured (Fig 4-9). Acoustical shadows are helpful in discriminating an occasional extension artifact from real bone. The measured femur length is then used to estimate gestational age from Table 4-1.

The humerus is equally accessible and equally precise in its correlation with gestational age.[7,12] The general shape and measurement technique are the same as for the femur. The humerus is often more freely mobile than the femur, arising from the lateral upper chest of the fetus. In cases in which the femur is not accessible (deep breech), the humerus is a fine alternative (see Table 4-1). Significant discrepancies between estimates of gestational age from long bone dimensions and head or menstrual estimates ought to raise the suspicion of some form of unexpected long bone dysplasia or dwarfism. A discrepancy of more than 2 weeks before 28 weeks' gestation or of 3 weeks after 28 weeks' gestation is significant.

Crown–Rump Measurement

The fetal crown–rump measurement or length (CRM or CRL) between 8 and 13 weeks' gestation is very closely related to gestational age. The observed variability of ±4 days (95% confidence) makes CRM a very accurate estimator of gestational age.[13]

Technique

In the pregnancy between 8 and 13 weeks' gestation, usually the whole gestation can be seen in one suprapubic field of view using a linear array realtime machine. The fetus will be seen within the sac, with heart action

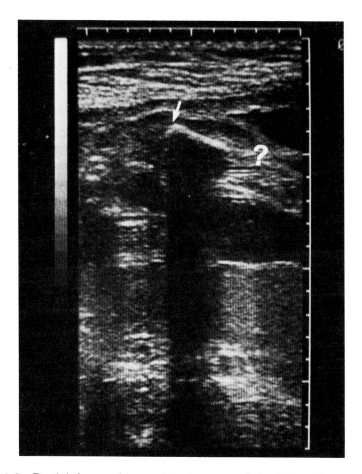

Fig 4-8. Partial femur. Incomplete images of fetal long bones often demonstrate a clear end point (arrow) at one end of the bone and a vague nonspecific landmark (?) at the other end. This vagueness to one landmark suggests incomplete capture of the bone.

and usually limb or trunk movement. Using both angular and rotational movement of the transducer, the operator must study the fetal mass and identify the longest fetal axis. Once the greatest long axis is found, the image is frozen and measured (Fig 4-10). The CRM should be repeated a minimum of three times to establish consistency, because fetal posturing and operator inaccuracy could lead to errors. In early pregnancy a full maternal bladder is helpful because it displaces the small bowel out of the pelvis and provides an acoustical window.

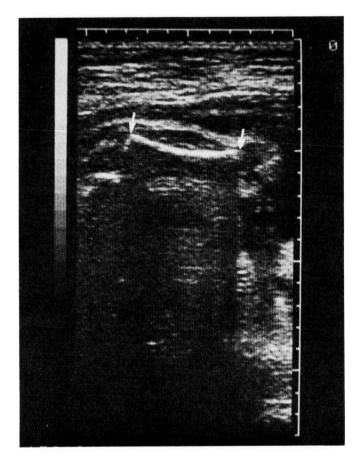

Fig 4-9. Complete femur. The complete femur illustrated here (arrows) demonstrates clear landmarks at each end, often with sharp shadowing, which may assist in identifying the end of the true bone.

A good practical estimate of gestational age will be produced by adding 6.5 to the CRM in centimeters to derive the gestational age in weeks (Table 4-2).[1]

Abdominal Circumference

Abdominal circumference is another fetal dimension that relates to gestational age.[8] It is a more difficult dimension to derive because correct

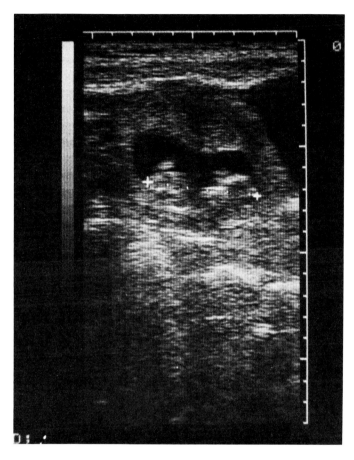

Fig 4-10. Crown–rump length. With rotation and angulation, the longest long axis of the fetal mass within the pregnant uterus may be captured, frozen, and measured.

imaging of the defined level of the fetal trunk can be complex. The technique involves aligning the scan plane with the fetal spine, then rotating 90° at the desired transverse level of the upper abdomen (Fig 4-11). The correct cephalocaudal position for the transverse scan to allow the abdominal circumference measurement is by convention where the umbilical vein is located within the liver mass (Fig 4-12). Once the approximate position is achieved, rotational movement of the transducer can be used to produce ideal side to side symmetry of the abdominal image, while an angling

Table 4-2. Crown–Rump Length

Estimated Gestational[1] Age (wks)	Length (mm)
8	17
8.5	20
9	24
9.5	28
10	33
10.5	38
11	43
11.5	49
12	55
12.5	61
13	68

movement may be used to normalize top to bottom image symmetry. It is important to maximize the sharpness of the distal fetal trunk surface to ensure proper position. Circumference may be estimated by either electronic or mechanical perimeter measurement or calculated from the mean of a long and short axis diameter. By either method, gestational age can then be estimated from Table 4-1. Due partly to the technical difficulty and greater variability, abdominal circumference is usually the last choice of possible dating dimensions but it may be useful to clarify discrepancies between other methods. Abdominal circumference is also used in the estimate of fetal weight, as we will see in later chapters.

Discrepancies and Averages

The BPD and the femur throughout pregnancy maintain a relatively constant relationship to one another and an approximately equivalent correlation to gestational age prior to 28 weeks' gestation. There is no statistical basis in any one fetus for choosing one over the other when a minor discrepancy within the expected range of variability of either dimension arises. Measuring multiple dating dimensions at every examination is recommended strongly and will serve at least two purposes. First, in pregnancies of less than 28 weeks, averaging the estimated gestational age from two or more measures appears to provide a more accurate estimate of age than single dimensional estimates.[2] In fact, some evidence suggests that the estimated date of confinement from the average of two or more such dimensions is superior to the last menstrual period in predicting onset of labor. A second benefit from using multiple dimensions is that a difference

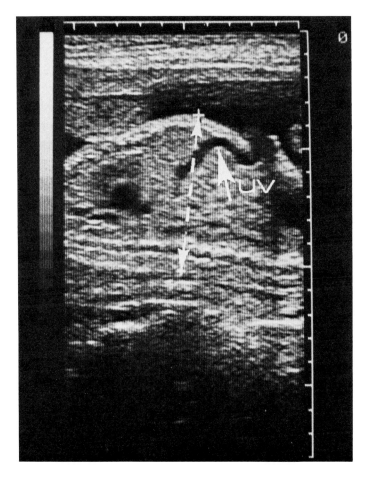

Fig 4-11. Level of abdominal circumference. This longitudinal midabdominal fetal scan illustrates the umbilical vein (uv) and the
level at which a transverse scan should be performed to
obtain an estimate of abdominal circumference. *Source:*
Reprinted with permission from *Obstetrics and Gynecology*
(1984;64), Copyright © 1984, Elsevier Science Publishing
Company, Inc.

of more than 2 weeks between the EGA derived from femur length and the
EGA derived from BPD (also head circumference or mean head diameter)
or abdominal circumference should lead to a critical reevaluation of both the
technique and the fetus. Either a serious technical error has been made in
one or more measurements or the fetus is significantly disproportionate.
Disproportionality might result from the cranial distortion already discussed

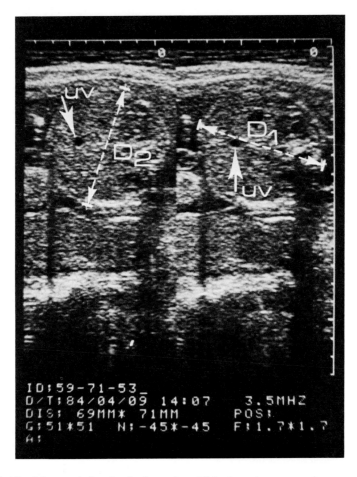

Fig 4-12. Mean abdominal diameter. This is a transverse scan at the level indicated in Figure 4-11. The umbilical vein (uv) should appear within the liver mass. Diameter one (D₁) and diameter two (D₂) are then measured and averaged to produce the mean abdominal diameter. *Source:* Reprinted with permission from *Obstetrics and Gynecology* (1984;64), Copyright © 1984, Elsevier Science Publishing Company, Inc.

or from unexpected dwarfism, microcephaly, or hydrocephalus. Measuring two or more fetal dimensions and comparing estimated age from each is, therefore, an important internal standard that every sonographer should use to check technique as well as to assess fetal growth.

If there is no option but to examine a fetus after 28 weeks' gestation, however, and a discrepancy is found, the age estimate from the femur or humerus length appears to be the most accurate available.

CLINICAL RECORDS

As in the case of any clinical technique, a clinician beginning an experience with sonographic dating should defer basing irreversible clinical decisions on ultrasound data until sufficient confidence is gained through practice and clinical correlation. Careful records should be kept and clinical outcome reviewed at intervals to assess the accuracy and precision of the process. These records may be kept easily in a log book dedicated to that purpose or on computer if one is available. If comparisons of sonographic and clinical gestational age reveal a consistent significant discrepancy, another dimensional growth chart may be chosen or the details of the technique reviewed and altered if necessary.

An appropriately circumspect approach will prevent clinical errors resulting from inexperience during the early part of a sonographic career.

REFERENCES

1. Bovicelli L, Orsini LF, Rizzo N, et al: Estimation of gestational age during the first trimester by realtime measurement of fetal crown-rump length and biparietal diameter. *J Clin Ultrasound* 9:71-75, 1981.

2. Hadlock FP, Deter RL, Harrist RB, et al: Computer assisted analysis of fetal age in the third trimester using multiple fetal growth parameters. *J Clin Ultrasound* 11:313-316, 1983.

3. Kopta MM, May RR, Crane JP: A comparison of the reliability of the estimated date of confinement predicted by crown-rump length and biparietal diameter. *Am J Obstet Gynecol* 145:562-565, 1983.

4. Kopta MM, Tomich PG, Crane JP: Ultrasonic methods of predicting the estimated date of confinement. *Obstet Gynecol* 57:657-660, 1981.

5. Sabbagha RE, Hughey M: Standardization of sonar cephalometry and gestational age. *Obstet Gynecol* 52:402-406, 1978.

6. Kurtz AB, Wapner RJ, Kurtz RJ, et al: Analysis of biparietal diameter as an accurate indicator of gestational age. *J Clin Ultrasound* 8:319-326, 1980.

7. Jeanty P, Rodesch F, Delbeke D, Dumont JE: Estimation of gestational age from measurements of fetal long bones. *J Ultrasound Med* 3:75-79, 1984.

8. Deter RL, Harrist RB, Hadlock FP, et al: Fetal head and abdominal circumferences: II. A critical re-evaluation of the relationship to menstrual age. *J Clin Ultrasound* 10:365–372, 1982.

9. Hill LM, Breckle R, Gehrking WC: The variable effects of oligohydramnios on the biparietal diameter and the cephalic index. *J Ultrasound Med* 3:93–95, 1984.

10. Wolfson RN, Zador IE, Halvorsen P, et al: Biparietal diameter in premature rupture of membranes: Errors in estimating gestational age. *J Clin Ultrasound* 11:371–374, 1983.

11. Hadlock FP, Harrist RB, Deter RL, et al: A prospective evaluation of fetal femur length as a predictor of gestational age. *J Ultrasound Med* 2:111–112, 1983.

12. Seeds JW, Cefalo RC: Relationship of fetal limb lengths to both biparietal diameter and gestational age. *Obstet Gynecol* 60:680–684, 1982.

13. O'Brien GD, Queenan JT, Campbell S: Assessment of gestational age in the second trimester by realtime ultrasound measurement of the femur length. *Am J Obstet Gynecol* 139:540–545, 1981.

14. Yeh MN, Bracero L, Reilly KB, et al: Ultrasonic measurement of the femur length as an index of fetal gestational age. *Am J Obstet Gynecol* 144:519–522, 1982.

Chapter 5

Evaluation of Fetal Growth

CLINICAL CONSIDERATIONS

The most commonly used definition of impaired fetal growth is a birth weight below the tenth percentile for gestational age, using birth weight standards representative of the clinical population.[1] By this definition, intrauterine growth retardation (IUGR) affects 10% of newborns. The clinical significance of IUGR includes a fourfold to eightfold increase in perinatal mortality and a 50% risk of neonatal morbidity.[2] Birth asphyxia, meconium aspiration pneumonia, polycythemia, hypoglycemia, and hypocalcemia are all recognized neonatal risks of the growth-impaired fetus.

Prenatal diagnosis should help reduce perinatal morbidity and mortality associated with IUGR, but diagnosis is complicated by the fact that a definition by birth weight alone identifies a population of small infants who are not uniform in appearance or clinical condition.[1] Infants with a birth weight below the tenth percentile for gestational age come from at least four categories of etiology (Fig 5-1). About 40% of these newborns are simply constitutionally small, with normal proportions. Their size is not the direct result of either fetal or maternal disease. About 10% of these newborns are small because of intrauterine infection. Rubella and cytomegalovirus infections are commonly reported. Another 10% are small because of genetic problems, such as trisomy 13 or 18, or renal agenesis (Potter's syndrome). The remaining 40% of newborns with a birth weight below the tenth percentile for gestational age are small because of a deprivational process secondary to chronic uteroplacental insufficiency.

The outcome for the infant whose growth is limited by progressive deprivation from maternal vascular disease or placental inadequacy is variable. The long-term outcome is good in the absence of birth asphyxia. These infants clearly might benefit from early detection, prenatal intensive care, and closely monitored labor and delivery. It is, therefore, the deprivational group toward whom most prenatal diagnostic efforts are directed.[3]

IUGR — ETIOLOGIES

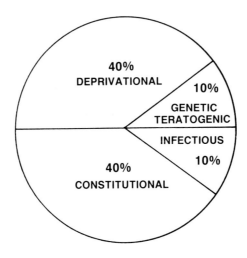

Fig 5-1. Causes of intrauterine growth retardation.

PRENATAL DIAGNOSIS

Clinical Suspicion

Traditionally, clinical diagnosis of IUGR has been poor, with as few as 50% of these infants detected and a false-positive diagnosis rate of up to 50%.[2] The curvilinear suprapubic fundal height measurement in centimeters, however, is a useful clinical screening tool (see Fig. 7-1).[4] When the fundal height is more than 4 cm below the gestational age in weeks, the probability of IUGR or a serious error in dating is as high as 90%. Clinical suspicion is also justified when maternal medical conditions are present that carry a high risk of IUGR, such as chronic hypertension, severe preeclampsia, chronic heart disease, or longstanding insulin-dependent diabetes. Pregnancies with a significant fundal growth lag or medical complications should benefit most from careful ultrasonic evaluation.

Ultrasonic Diagnosis

The ultrasonic diagnosis of growth impairment is based on the technical ability to measure fetal dimensions. The normal patterns of growth of such dimensions are recorded from reference populations of normal pregnancies delivering non-growth-impaired infants, and by comparison to these normal values, a deviation may be detected.[3,5-9] Furthermore, chronic deprivation can result in alterations of fetal function such as urine output, and the resulting oligohydramnios may be observed with ultrasound.[10-12] Technical precision of fetal ultrasound measurement continues to exceed the clinical accuracy in predicting IUGR. Part of the reason for inaccuracy is that all dimensional growth curves are necessarily based on gestational age, and an accurate gestational age is not always known. Also, not all fetal dimensions are equally reduced in cases of impaired fetal growth. It appears most appropriate that a combination of both clinical and biophysical data be used in the diagnosis and care of pregnancies complicated by IUGR to achieve optimal results.

Biparietal Diameter

The use of biparietal diameter (BPD) to diagnose IUGR has been shown to detect only about 50% of affected infants.[9] This may in part result from poor clinical dating but may also be the result of an asymmetry of fetal growth in many cases.[5,9] A major fetal adaption to acute or chronic deprivation is a redistribution of cardiac output favoring the heart, brain, and adrenal circulation at the expense of the trunk, limbs, and notably the renal blood flow.[1] Such an adaption preserves brain and cranial growth later into the process. Liver mass is especially severely restricted. The anthropomorphic result is an infant whose weight and abdominal circumference are below the tenth percentile for gestational age but whose cranium and BPD are not proportionately reduced. BPD is, therefore, an insensitive indicator of deprivational IUGR. BPD is reduced in cases of symmetrical IUGR as a result of constitutional, infectious, or genetic causes. A longstanding or severe deprivational process will finally lead to a reduction of brain and cranial growth. Such a pattern of biparietal growth has been described as a "late flattening" type.

The disproportionate affectation of head and abdomen produces an asymmetry in fetal dimensions characteristic of deprivational IUGR at some point in the deprivational sequence even though at delivery the infant might appear more symmetrical.

Abdominal Circumference

Since fetal trunk dimensions are reduced in all types of IUGR, it is not surprising that most evidence suggests that the abdominal circumference is the most useful single sonographic dimension in detecting IUGR.[6,9] The reported accuracy exceeds 80%. Furthermore, the ratio of head circumference to abdominal circumference follows a predictable pattern during normal pregnancy and reflects the symmetry of fetal growth. The detection of an anomaly of this relationship not only allows the diagnosis of IUGR but also, by assessing symmetry, gives some insight into the probable cause.

Abdominal circumference is measured exactly as described in Chapter 4 (see Figs 4-11 and 4-12). If the mean diameter method is used, then growth curves are easily reduced to the mean abdominal diameter for a given gestational age since this value is a fixed mathematical relative of the abdominal circumference. Head circumference may be measured in the same ways, and comparison of circumferences may be reduced to a comparison of mean diameters for the assessment of symmetry. To assess symmetry, the mean head diameter is divided by the mean abdominal diameter and the resultant ratio is compared with the values in Table 5-1.[13,14] A ratio above 2 standard deviations (SD) above the mean for gestational age would suggest significant asymmetry and support a diagnosis of IUGR.

Table 5-1. Normal Mean Head to Abdomen Diameter Ratios

Gestational Age (wks)	−2 SD	Mean Head Diameter/ Mean Abdominal Diameter	+2 SD
20	1.06	1.15	1.24
21	1.05	1.14	1.24
22	1.04	1.13	1.23
23	1.03	1.12	1.22
24	1.02	1.12	1.21
25	1.01	1.11	1.20
26	1.00	1.10	1.19
27	1.00	1.09	1.18
28	0.99	1.08	1.18
29	0.98	1.07	1.17
30	0.97	1.07	1.16
31	0.96	1.06	1.15
32	0.95	1.05	1.14
33	0.95	1.04	1.13
34	0.94	1.03	1.13
35	0.93	1.02	1.12
36	0.92	1.01	1.11
37	0.91	1.01	1.10
38	0.90	1.00	1.09
39	0.89	0.99	1.08
40	0.89	0.98	1.08

Source: Adapted with permission from *American Journal of Roentgenology* (1982;139), Copyright © 1982, Williams & Wilkins Company.

Amniotic Fluid Volume

As mentioned before, a functional corollary of deprivational growth retardation is decreased fetal renal blood flow and urine output. Ultrasonic studies of bladder filling rates in growth-impaired fetuses have confirmed decreased output. The strong association of oligohydramnios with IUGR is further supportive evidence of decreased urine production in these cases and results from the redistribution of cardiac output. The sonographic diagnosis of oligohydramnios is, however, relatively subjective. Precise determination of amniotic fluid volume is difficult. Manning and colleagues defined oligohydramnios as the absence of at least a pocket of amniotic fluid with a 1-cm greatest dimension and found IUGR in 90% of cases lacking this minimum.[11] In 94% of cases with at least a 1-cm pocket, birth weight was above the tenth percentile.[11] Other authors recommend a slightly less restrictive definition.[10,12] The subjective assessment of relative amniotic fluid volume is a skill developed after some experience with realtime ultrasound. The sonographer will develop a sensitivity to amniotic fluid volume, and a deficiency will become apparent even before it is reduced to less than a single pocket of 1-cm diameter. It is appropriate to suspect IUGR whenever unexpected oligohydramnios is found with crowding of fetal small parts and poor visual outline of a fetal trunk in contact with the uterine wall throughout the uterus.

Estimated Fetal Weight

As we will see in greater detail in Chapter 6, fetal weight may be estimated from combinations of fetal dimensions such as BPD and abdominal circumference. Although the techniques serve a wide variety of applications, the use of sonographic estimated fetal weight specifically for the diagnosis of IUGR has been investigated and found to detect up to 90% of affected infants.[3] This is probably somewhat due to the fact that most weight estimation methods are based in part on abdominal circumference, which is a sensitive parameter of fetal growth. An estimated fetal weight may be compared with normal values in Table 5-2.[15]

Total Intrauterine Volume

Since the total intrauterine volume (TIUV) represents the composite aggregate of fetus, fluid, and placenta, and since all of these components are diminished with IUGR, it is appropriate to assume that accurate estimation of TIUV would be a sensitive indicator of impaired fetal growth. The method requires the use of a static contact ultrasound machine to measure the greatest length, greatest depth, and the greatest width of the uterus,

Table 5-2. Range of Estimated Fetal Weights in Grams

EGA (wks)	5th	50th	95th
25	608	749	922
26	703	865	1064
27	806	992	1221
28	918	1130	1391
29	1038	1278	1573
30	1166	1435	1766
31	1299	1599	1968
32	1436	1768	2177
33	1576	1940	2388
34	1715	2111	2599
35	1851	2279	2806
36	1982	2440	3005
37	2103	2590	3191
38	2211	2726	3360
39	2304	2843	3508
40	2377	2939	3633

Source: Adapted with permission from *Journal of Ultrasound in Medicine* (1984;3), Copyright © 1984, WB Saunders Company.

including placenta. These three dimensions are multiplied together and the product factored by 0.5233 to obtain an estimate of TIUV. Although early reports indicated a high degree of accuracy at predicting IUGR if the TIUV was reduced below 1.5 standard deviations below the mean for gestational age, further experience has found an impractical degree of technical variability that diminishes the utility of TIUV in clinical practice.[16-19]

Unsure Dates

All of the techniques mentioned so far require knowledge of gestational age. Inaccurate dates would result in inaccuracies in the assessment of the dimension. Yet not all high-risk pregnancies allow accurate clinical dating. It is, therefore, useful early in the prenatal course of known high-risk pregnancies to obtain ultrasonic assignment or confirmation of gestational dates to allow for the future assessment of the quality of fetal growth. Many patients, however, register late, when such sonographic data may be less accurate or already affected by the impairment process. When IUGR is suspected in such a pregnancy with poor clinical dates or late registry, the rate of interval growth becomes an important diagnostic indicator. Assessment of growth rate requires at least two examinations separated by a minimum of 2 weeks. BPD or mean head diameter, abdominal circumference or mean abdominal diameter, femur length, and estimated weight should be recorded. During the interval between examinations, antepartum fetal heart rate testing may be prudent to monitor fetal condition. Expected growth rates of BPD and abdominal circumference or mean abdominal diameter may be estimated, as well as the expected fetal weight gain (Table 5-3). A normal or near normal growth rate during the interval suggests the possibility of incorrect dates.

An indicator of fetal condition that is relatively independent of gestational age is the visual assessment of amniotic fluid volume. An adequate amniotic fluid volume is reassuring that the fetus under examination may not be growth impaired on a uteroplacental insufficiency basis or at least is not in imminent danger.

Mean Abdominal Diameter/Femur Length

The relationship of abdominal circumference and mean diameter to femur length follows a predictable course throughout pregnancy. The detection of an abnormality of this relationship would suggest an impairment of fetal soft tissue growth indicative of deprivation. Furthermore, the detection of an anomaly of this relationship would not require a precise knowledge of gestational age. Early studies of both abdominal circumference and mean abdominal diameter related to femur length do show a diagnostic value in these methods but do not yet show sensitivity or accuracy in the diagnosis of IUGR superior to abdominal circumference alone. It remains possible,

Table 5-3. Expected Interval Growth After 2-Week Interval

Gestational Age (wks)	Biparietal Diameter (mm)	Femur Length (mm)	Humerus Length (mm)	Mean Head Diameter (mm)	Mean Abdominal Diameter (mm)	Estimated Fetal Weight (g)
25	6	5	4	6	7	243
26	5	5	4	6	6	265
27	5	5	4	6	7	286
28	6	5	4	6	7	305
29	5	5	4	6	6	321
30	4	4	3	6	6	333
31	5	5	3	5	6	341
32	5	5	4	4	7	343
33	3	4	3	4	6	339
34	3	4	3	4	5	329
35	4	5	3	4	6	311
36	3	5	3	4	6	286
37	2	4	3	4	6	253
38	2	4	3	3	6	213

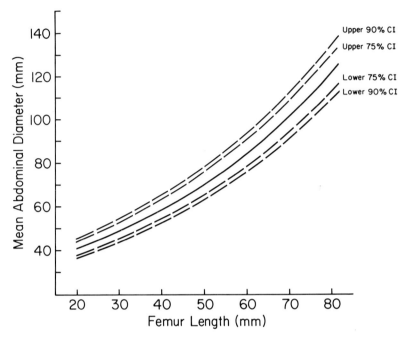

Fig 5-2. Mean abdominal diameter—femur length. Normal relationship between mean abdominal diameter and femur length in normal pregnancy. A mean abdominal diameter falling below the lower 75% confidence interval (CI) for a measured femur length suggests the possibility of deprivational growth retardation.

Table 5-4. Biophysical Profile

Observation	Score	
	2 Points	*0 Points*
Fetal breathing movements	30 Second per 30-minute interval	Absent
Trunk movements	3 Movements per 30-minute interval	Absent
Limb movements	Present	Absent
Nonstress test	Reactive	Nonreactive
Amniotic fluid	1-cm pocket or more	No 1-cm pocket

Source: Adapted with permission from *American Journal of Obstetrics and Gynecology* (1981;140), Copyright © 1981, CV Mosby Company.

however, that mean abdominal diameter to femur length ratio abnormalities specifically indicate growth impairment for deprivational reasons (Fig 5-2).

Diagnostic Summary

The sensitive prenatal diagnosis of IUGR requires careful clinical attention to measurement of fundal height and attention to clinical presence of maternal medical conditions associated with impaired fetal growth. When IUGR is suspected, sonographic evaluation of BPD, mean head diameter, abdominal circumference or mean abdominal diameter, femur length, amniotic fluid volume, and estimated fetal weight offer the clinician an objective data base for accurate diagnosis. Serial examinations are usually necessary.

Clinical Surveillance

If IUGR is diagnosed, ultrasound may also be a valuable tool in the follow-up of the pregnancy. The diagnosis of IUGR is not by itself sufficient justification for delivery prior to fetal maturity. Delivery is indicated only when maturity is assured or when direct evidence of fetal distress is developed. The serial sonographic observation of fetal limb movements, trunk movements, breathing movements, and amniotic fluid volume, combined with nonstress fetal heart rate monitoring has been proposed as a "biophysical profile."[20-23] Such an evaluation has been shown to be very sensitive to fetal condition (Table 5-4). Two points are awarded for each normal observation, with 10 as the maximum score if all five functions are noted to be normal. A score of 8 or 10 is repeated in 1 week. A score of 4 or 6 is repeated within 24 hours. A score of 2 or 0 indicates fetal distress, and such a pregnancy should be evaluated for delivery.

REFERENCES

1. Seeds JW: Impaired fetal growth: Definition and clinical diagnosis. *Obstet Gynecol* 64:303–310, 1984.

2. Galbraith RS, Karchmar EJ, Piercy WN, et al: The clinical prediction of intrauterine growth retardation. *Am J Obstet Gynecol* 133:281, 1979.

3. Seeds JW: Impaired fetal growth: Ultrasonic evaluation and clinical management. *Obstet Gynecol* 64:577–584, 1984.

4. Belizan JM, Villar J, Nardin JC, et al: Diagnosis of intrauterine growth retardation by a simple clinical method: Measurement of uterine height. *Am J Obstet Gynecol* 131:643, 1978.

5. Crane JP, Kopta MM: Prediction of intrauterine growth retardation via ultrasonically measured head/abdominal circumference ratios. *Obstet Gynecol* 54:597–601, 1979.

6. Deter RL, Harrist RB, Hadlock FP, et al: The use of ultrasound in the detection of intrauterine growth retardation: A review. *J Clin Ultrasound* 10:9–16, 1982.

7. Ott WJ: The use of ultrasonic fetal head circumference for predicting expected date of confinement. *J Clin Ultrasound* 12:411–415, 1984.

8. Queenan JT, Kubarych SF, Cook LN, et al: Diagnostic ultrasound for detection of intrauterine growth retardation. *Am J Obstet Gynecol* 124:865–873, 1976.

9. Wittmann BK, Robinson HP, Aitchison T, et al: The value of diagnostic ultrasound as a screening test for intrauterine growth retardation: Comparison of nine parameters. *Am J Obstet Gynecol* 134:30–35, 1979.

10. Gross TL, Sokol RJ, Wilson MV, et al: Using ultrasound and amniotic fluid determinations to diagnose intrauterine growth retardation before birth: A clinical method. *Am J Obstet Gynecol* 143:265, 1982.

11. Manning FA, Hill LM, Platt LD: Qualitative amniotic fluid volume determination by ultrasound: Antepartum detection of intrauterine growth retardation. *Am J Obstet Gynecol* 139:254–258, 1981.

12. Philipson EH, Sokol RJ, Williams T: Oligohydramnios: Clinical associations and predictive value for intrauterine growth retardation. *Am J Obstet Gynecol* 146:271–278, 1983.

13. Hadlock FP, Deter RL, Harrist RB: Fetal abdominal circumference as a predictor of menstrual age. *AJR* 139:367–370, 1982.

14. Hadlock FP, Deter RL, Harrist RB: Fetal head circumference: Relation to menstrual age. *AJR* 138:649–653, 1982.

15. Jeanty P, Cantraine F, Romero R, et al: A longitudinal study of fetal weight growth. *J Ultrasound Med* 3:321–328, 1984.

16. Chinn DH, Filly RA, Callen PW: Prediction of intrauterine growth retardation by sonographic estimation of total intrauterine volume. *J Clin Ultrasound* 9:175–179, 1981.

17. Grossman M, Flynn JJ, Aufrichtig D, et al: Pitfalls in ultrasonic determination of total intrauterine volume. *J Clin Ultrasound* 10:17–20, 1982.

18. Kurtz AB, Shaw WM, Kurtz RJ, et al: The inaccuracy of total uterine volume measurements: Sources of error and a proposed solution. *J Ultrasound Med* 3:289–297, 1984.

19. Levine SC, Filly RA, Creasy RK: Identification of fetal growth retardation by ultrasonographic estimation of total intrauterine volume. *J Clin Ultrasound* 7:21–26, 1979.

20. Baskett TF, Gray JH, Prewett SJ, et al: Antepartum fetal assessment using a fetal biophysical profile score. *Am J Obstet Gynecol* 148:630, 1984.

21. Manning FA, Baskett TF, Morrison I, et al: Fetal biophysical profile scoring: A prospective study in 1,184 high-risk patients. *Am J Obstet Gynecol* 140:289–294, 1981.

22. Manning FA, Lange IR, Morrison I, et al: Fetal biophysical profile score and the nonstress test: A comparative trial. *Obstet Gynecol* 64:326–331, 1984.

23. Schifrin BS, Guntes V, Gergely RC, et al: The role of realtime scanning in antenatal fetal surveillance. *Am J Obstet Gynecol* 140:525–530, 1981.

Chapter 6

Ultrasonic Estimation of
Fetal Weight

CLINICAL CONSIDERATIONS

An accurate estimate of fetal weight facilitates a wide variety of obstetrical decisions.[1] In pregnancies complicated by a medical condition that often requires preterm delivery, fetal weight may be the only objective parameter available that correlates with neonatal survival. Premature labor, premature rupture of fetal membranes, and fetal malpresentation are clinical circumstances that are better managed with an accurate estimate of fetal weight. Decisions regarding mode of delivery, necessity for referral, aggressiveness of resuscitation, and the role of intrapartum fetal heart rate monitoring are often made on the basis of an estimate of neonatal survival. Although evidence supports gestational age as a better predictor of fetal survivability, an accurate gestational age is unknown in many cases and, therefore, an accurate estimate of fetal weight becomes the next best objective indicator of neonatal prognosis. Between 25 and 30 weeks' gestation, survival is shown to be strongly influenced by the attending physician's prospective estimate of survival.[1] If neonatal survival is expected, a clinician is more likely to monitor a fetus in labor, perform a cesarean delivery for fetal indications, or refer a pregnant patient for delivery near a neonatal intensive care unit.

Manual estimation of fetal weight has well-known limitations. Manual estimates are most accurate when the fetus is near average size at term. Inaccuracy in manual estimates grows progressively as extremes of low birth weight or macrosomia are observed. Specifically, in the low birth weight infant, manual estimation of fetal weight consistently demonstrates substantial error.[2] Management decisions based only on manual estimates of fetal weight, therefore, necessarily involve a significant risk of error. Assuming a viable child to be nonviable and contributing to perinatal death by choice of birth method or by failure to provide aggressive perinatal care

79

might be the most tragic possibility. However, the performance of an unnecessary cesarean delivery of an infant too immature to survive is an equally unsatisfying outcome owing to inaccurate assessment of fetal viability. Therefore, an accurate estimate of fetal weight can significantly aid in the care of the complicated pregnancy.

ULTRASONIC METHODS

The basis for the sonographic estimation of fetal weight is simple. Fetal mass is related to fetal dimensions. Accurate assessment of a combination of fetal dimensions and careful correlation of these with the observed birth weight of a known reference population should generate a data base capable of predicting birth weight.

If all fetuses were perfectly symmetrical and identical in proportions, only one dimension would be needed, and it could be any dimension. Since all fetuses are not identical nor perfectly symmetrical, the history of sonographic estimation of fetal weight has been a search for the perfect dimension or set of dimensions that most accurately predicts fetal weight with minimal error and that is within the practical skills of most sonographers.

Early in the evolution of ultrasonic estimation of fetal weight, Campbell reported the relationship of abdominal circumference to birth weight with a reported error of $\pm 9.1\%$ of 91 g/kg.[3] The cases in his series were uncomplicated, however, and no serious pathologic condition was reported among the infants. Therefore, although his level of precision was good, application of the method to a high-risk population with the possibility of IUGR and anthropomorphic asymmetry is possibly inappropriate. Furthermore, his dimensional data were derived from a contact static ultrasound machine calibrated at a speed of sound in soft tissue of 1500 meters per second, and the dimensions, therefore, would not correlate exactly with data from contemporary realtime equipment.

Other investigators have since proposed that the use of a combination of more than one fetal dimension would reflect a measure of the symmetry of fetal growth in the estimate of fetal weight. Systems have included biparietal diameter, abdominal circumference or mean abdominal diameter, femur length, thigh circumference, and even serial sequenced tomograms of the fetus with computer analysis to provide an aggregate estimate of fetal volume as the basis for weight estimation. Accuracy of the reported methods has varied, but most methods demonstrate error of about $\pm 10\%$ or about 100 g/kg (1 SD). Most recent methods involve the ultrasonic measurement of either abdominal circumference or mean abdominal diameter and of biparietal diameter. Table 6-1 lists four selected fetal weight estimation formulae for consideration based on these fetal dimensions.[4-7]

Warsof and co-workers, in 1977, reported a method for the estimation of fetal weight using abdominal circumference and biparietal diameter with a reported accuracy of ±10.6% (106 g/kg) for 1 standard deviation (SD). Their formula (equation 1 in Table 6-1) was based on data from 85 infants.[4] The technique has since been evaluated by other investigators, and the original reported accuracy has been confirmed. It is remarkable that several observers have found even greater accuracy in the infant weighing less than 1500 g, since only 12 of the original 85 reference infants weighed under 1500 g.[8,9] Table 6-2 gives estimated fetal weights based on equation 1.

Equation 2 was developed from the same data base as equation 1, in the same ultrasound unit. It was evaluated prospectively, and the mean error was reported to be slightly smaller. In comparative evaluations by other authors, however, no clear superiority has been shown for either formula.[8]

Thurnau and colleagues developed equation 3, and Weinberger and his associates proposed equation 4 for the estimation of fetal weights specifically in the case of the fetus weighing less than 2000 g.[6,7] Both of these equations are linear and do not involve logarithmic transformations and, therefore, might be easier to apply in practice. A comparative evaluation of relative accuracies of these four methods is found in Table 6-3 and appears to show that equation 4 offers estimates of fetal weight in the small infant with the lowest error.[7]

The practical choice of specific method remains with the individual. These are only four of the many available techniques, selected here for both proven level of accuracy and practical applicability. They are all clearly superior to manual estimation of fetal weight. When beginning the practice of weight estimation, each operator is advised to record and collect dimensional data from his or her own practice and evaluate all of these methods and others before finally choosing one. Continued careful record keeping would allow interval reevaluation of accuracy.

TECHNIQUE

All of the techniques considered here use some measure of cranial mass, such as biparietal diameter, and a measure of somatic mass, such as abdominal circumference or mean abdominal diameter.

Table 6-1. Fetal Weight Estimation Formulae

1. $Log(BW) = 1.599 + 0.144(BPD) + 0.032(AC) - 0.111(BPD^2 \times AC)/1000$
2. $Log(BW) = 1.7492 + 0.166(BPD) + 0.046(AC) - 2.646(AC \times BPD^2)/1000$
3. $BW = -299.076 + 9.337(BPD \times AC)$
4. $BW = 10.1(AC \times BPD) - 481$

Key: BW, birth weight; BPD, biparietal diameter; AC, abdominal circumference.

Table 6-2. Fetal Weight Estimation (g)

Abdominal Circumference (cm)		17.0	18.0	19.0	20.0	21.0	22.0
Mean Abdominal Diameter (cm)		5.4	5.7	6.0	6.4	6.7	7.0
Femur Length (mm)	Biparietal Diameter (mm)						
37	55	478	511	546	583	622	665
39	57	506	540	577	616	657	702
40	59	535	571	609	650	694	740
42	61	566	604	644	686	732	780
44	63	598	638	679	724	772	822
46	65	632	673	717	764	813	866
48	67	668	711	757	805	857	912
49	69	705	750	798	848	902	960
52	71	745	791	841	894	950	1009
54	73	786	835	886	941	999	1061
55	75	829	880	934	991	1051	1115
56	77	874	927	983	1042	1105	1172
59	79	922	977	1035	1096	1161	1230
61	81	971	1028	1088	1152	1220	1291
63	83	1023	1082	1145	1177	1211	1355
64	85	1078	1139	1203	1272	1344	1420
67	87	1134	1198	1265	1335	1410	1489
70	89	1194	1259	1329	1402	1478	1560
72	91	1256	1324	1395	1470	1550	1633

Biparietal Diameter

The biparietal diameter used in all of the methods considered here is measured in the same fashion as for gestational age assignment. This is the largest fetal cranial diameter, leading edge of skull table to leading edge of skull table, perpendicular to the midline of the cranial oval outline in an occipitofrontal scan plane at the level of the cavum septum pellucidum and the thalami (see Fig 4-4).

Femur Length

When the biparietal diameter is distorted by compression, as in the case of oligohydramnios, or is unavailable due to deep pelvic engagement, femur length can be a reasonable substitute.[10] This is based on the close linear relationship between femur length and biparietal diameter. Table 6-2 is, therefore, formatted with both biparietal diameter and the appropriate corresponding femur length. The femur is measured as described in Chapter 4, as the longest dimension of the continuous bone parallel to the shaft (see

23.0	24.0	25.0	26.0	27.0	28.0	29.0	30.0
7.3	7.6	8.0	8.3	8.6	8.9	9.2	9.6
710	759	811	866	925	988	1055	1127
749	800	854	912	973	1039	1109	1184
790	843	899	959	1023	1092	1165	1243
832	887	946	1009	1076	1147	1223	1304
876	934	995	1060	1130	1204	1283	1367
922	982	1046	1114	1186	1263	1345	1433
970	1033	1099	1170	1245	1325	1410	1500
1021	1085	1154	1227	1305	1388	1476	1570
1073	1140	1212	1287	1368	1454	1545	1642
1127	1197	1271	1350	1433	1522	1616	1716
1184	1256	1333	1414	1501	1592	1690	1793
1242	1317	1397	1481	1570	1665	1765	1872
1303	1381	1463	1550	1642	1740	1843	1953
1367	1447	1532	1621	1716	1817	1923	2036
1433	1515	1603	1695	1793	1897	2006	2122
1501	1586	1676	1772	1872	1978	2091	2210
1572	1660	1752	1850	1954	2063	2178	2300
1645	1736	1831	1931	2037	2149	2267	2392
1721	1814	1912	2015	2124	2238	2359	2486

Source: Adapted with permission from *American Journal of Obstetrics and Gynecology* (1977;128), Copyright © 1977, CV Mosby Company.

Fig 4-9). Femur length is then used in the estimation of fetal weight from Table 6-2 in the same way that biparietal diameter would be used.

Table 6-3. Evaluation of Relative Accuracies of Four Fetal Weight Estimation Formulae

	%Cases with Error Under:	
Equation	10%	20%
1	68.2%	92.7%
2	63.4%	97.5%
3	56.0%	87.8%
4	78.0%	95.1%

Source: Adapted with permission from *American Journal of Roentgenology* (1984;141), Copyright ©, Williams & Wilkins Company.

Abdominal Circumference

The abdominal circumference is estimated from a transverse image of the fetal abdomen, perpendicular to the spine at a level just below the fetal diaphragm where a short segment of the umbilical vein may be seen within the liver mass (see Figs 4-11 and 4-12). The scan plane must be carefully chosen to achieve as close to perfect perpendicularity as possible. Being off an axis in any direction would introduce a positive error in estimating circumference. Choosing a scan plane closer to the caudal pole of the fetus would introduce a negative error as the abdomen is somewhat smaller closer to the umbilicus.

The transducer should be aligned with the fetal spine, and at the level of the upper abdomen, turned 90°. A sliding movement may then be used to approach the desired level where the umbilical vein is seen, not just under the anterior abdominal wall but deep in the liver mass. At this level, a rotational movement of the transducer is used to optimize symmetry of the trunk section from side to side and an angling movement is used to maximize sharpness of the distal fetal skin surface. When maximum side to side symmetry and optimal distal surface sharpness are achieved at a level where the umbilical vein is seen opposite the spine within the liver mass, the image is frozen and measured. At least three, and preferably five, such images should be composed and measured.

The circumference of the abdomen imaged by the above technique may be estimated in one of two ways. The perimeter of the abdominal image may be measured using either electronic or mechanical means. Many contemporary machines incorporate some electronic perimeter system for circumference assessment. If such a device is not available, a Polaroid photograph may be taken and a mechanical map reader may be rolled along the perimeter of the abdomen and then run out along the marginal scale to estimate circumference. In both cases, considerable positive error may be introduced by irregularities in following the outline of the abdomen. Alternatively, two perpendicular diameters of the abdominal image measured on screen electronically may be averaged and either used directly or multiplied by 3.1416 to produce an estimate of circumference, as described in Chapter 4.

Perimeter measurement requires precise fidelity to the edge of the abdomen throughout the entire process. There are few operators who would not deviate from the true path with either electronic or mechanical perimeter measurement systems. The use of the mean abdominal diameter from a carefully composed image is more practical and reproducible than perimeter measurement.[7,9] An inappropriate image, either at the wrong level or at the wrong angle, has the potential for introducing error of much greater magnitude than the error introduced by the method of measurement of the image once composed.

Table 6-2 is constructed with both abdominal circumference and mean abdominal diameter to allow weight estimation regardless of the measurement method preferred.

Clinical Accuracy

The correlation between estimated fetal weight and actual fetal weight is not perfect. Although clearly superior to clinical methods, all of the techniques presented here provide a result with 67% (1 SD) confidence that the estimate will be within 10% of the actual birth weight and with 95% (2 SD) confidence that the estimate will be within 20% of the birth weight. This estimated risk of error must be considered in clinical management based on a sonographic estimate of fetal weight.

REFERENCES

1. Paul RH, Koh KS, Monfared AH: Obstetric factors influencing outcome in infants weighing from 1001 to 1500 grams. *Am J Obstet Gynecol* 133:503–508, 1979.
2. Loeffler FE: Clinical foetal weight prediction. *J Obstet Gynaecol Br Commonw* 79:675–679, 1967.
3. Campbell S, Wilkin D: Ultrasound measurement of fetal abdominal circumference in estimation of fetal weight. *Br J Obstet Gynaecol* 82:689–693, 1975.
4. Warsof SL, Gohar P, Berkowitz RL, et al: The estimation of fetal weight by computer assisted analysis. *Am J Obstet Gynecol* 128:881–892, 1977.
5. Shephard MJ, Richards VA, Berkowitz RL, et al: An evaluation of two equations for predicting fetal weight by ultrasound. *Am J Obstet Gynecol* 142:47–54, 1982.
6. Thurnau GR, Tamura RK, Sabbagha R: A simple estimated fetal weight based on realtime ultrasound measurements of fetuses less than 34 weeks' gestation. *Am J Obstet Gynecol* 145:557–561, 1983.
7. Weinberger E, Cyr DR, Hirsh JH, et al: Estimating fetal weights less than 2000 grams: An accurate and simple method. *AJR* 141:973–977, 1984.
8. Key TC, Dattel BJ, Resnick R: The ultrasonographic estimation of fetal weight in the very low birthweight infant. *Am J Obstet Gynecol* 145:574–578, 1983.
9. Ott WJ: Clinical application of fetal weight determination by realtime ultrasound measurements. *Obstet Gynecol* 57:758–762, 1981.
10. Seeds JW, Cefalo RC, Bowes WA: Femur length in the estimation of fetal weight less than 1500 grams. *Am J Obstet Gynecol* 149:233–235, 1984.

Chapter 7

Prenatal Diagnosis: Clinical Considerations

Four to 6% of all infants are born with some malformation. Roughly half of these are minor, but the remainder are of major significance and many are lethal deformities. Techniques now available for prenatal diagnosis of many of these defects include ultrasound, amniotic fluid or maternal serum α-fetoprotein assessment, cytogenetic analysis of cultured amniotic fluid cells or chorionic villus biopsy material, amniotic fluid analysis for byproducts of defective enzyme systems, fetoscopy with or without fetal blood sampling, and restriction endonuclease analysis of chromatin material obtained from amniotic fluid cells.

The prenatal diagnosis of a birth defect early in gestation allows parental consideration of pregnancy termination or preparation by the family for the birth of the child with special needs or disabilities. Furthermore, prenatal diagnosis allows, in selected cases, consideration of prenatal therapeutic intervention, such as drainage of an obstructed organ or indwelling diversion drainage of an obstructed system. Prenatal diagnosis also encourages referral in utero for birth at a perinatal center that is equipped and prepared for the immediate neonatal care of the infant. Even extensive neonatal support cannot prevent all perinatal losses due to malformation, but there are many examples of infants whose survival was directly aided by prior knowledge of the malformation and preparation for birth.

Prenatal diagnosis is a general process that includes many technologies directed at the detection usually of specific lesions or conditions. The specificity of many of these methods requires some knowledge of the type of defect for which the fetus in question is at risk. Some of these methods are completely safe, while others carry some small risk. There is a progression in risk from ultrasound to radiography to amniocentesis to chorionic villus sampling to fetoscopy, and a parallel progression in the specificity of the tests from the more general fetal physical examination available with ultrasound to the more specific fetal blood sampling for biochemical analysis or karyotype. So far ultrasound is without evidence of direct risk to human pregnancy, although it is not yet proven safe beyond all doubt. Radiographic methods involve low risk at very low absorbed dosages, but the significance of the rare childhood cancers that might result from even small dosages demands extreme care in the use of ionizing radiation for prenatal diagnosis. The procedure-related risk of amniocentesis has been placed at 0.25% to 0.50%. This represents excess pregnancy losses above the rate of loss seen at comparable gestational ages without amniocentesis. Chorionic villus sampling appears to introduce a risk of excess loss of about 2%. Fetoscopy even in the most experienced hands appears to carry a risk of excess loss of 4% to 5%.

MALFORMATIONS: ETIOLOGIES

Human birth defects are the result of a variety of factors. In over half of the cases the specific cause remains unknown. In about 10% of malformations, the cause is believed to be environmental, that is, the result of maternal drug ingestion, fever, or physical compromise of the intrauterine environment. From 10% to 20% of congenital disease is inherited according to mendelian principles of inheritance, such as autosomal dominant, autosomal recessive, or sex-linked recessive patterns of transmission.

The majority of congenital malformations with a genetic basis occur as the result of a combination of factors, or as the composite result of several related genes. These malformations typically involve a single organ system and include such lesions as cleft lip or palate, neural tube defects, many obstructive lesions of the urinary tract, and the majority of congenital heart lesions. These malformations are called multifactorial or polygenic in origin. It is this category of congenital malformations from which a large number of defects detectable with ultrasound come.

PRENATAL DIAGNOSIS: INDICATIONS

Clinical History

The majority of children with birth defects are born to women with no history and often with no clinical indications for referral for prenatal diagnosis. Certain groups, however, may be identified by virtue of previous history, age, or ethnic origin as being at increased risk for congenital disease in their offspring, and these groups can be offered prenatal or preconceptional screening. Preconceptional carrier testing of couples of Eastern European Jewish ancestry for Tay-Sachs disease is an example. A family history of hemophilia should lead to preconceptional carrier testing or risk assessment. Cytogenetic diagnosis is often offered to women who have experienced multiple miscarriages and/or the birth of a child with malformations. Autosomal translocations may be found in a clinically normal parent carrier who is at increased risk of unbalanced progeny and possibly repeated abortion.

The largest number of referrals for prenatal diagnosis are made because of increased maternal age. The risk of fetal aneuploidy (any departure from the normal 46:XX or 46:XY karyotype) rises with maternal and, later, with paternal age. The risk of aneuploidy for a woman who is 35 to 36 years old at the birth of her child is about 1.3%. About half of these abnormalities take the form of trisomy 21 or Down syndrome. The risk of all aneuploidy, including Down syndrome, continues to rise thereafter. Although there remains some variation, most authorities agree that it is appropriate to offer prenatal cytogenetic diagnosis to any couple when the mother will be 35 years old at delivery or when the father is over 55. This does not mean the couple must undergo prenatal diagnosis. It means that prenatal diagnosis should be offered to them and the risks and significance of affectation and the risks of the procedure explained. The discussion should be documented in the hospital chart and their decision noted.

Recognized indications for prenatal diagnosis are summarized in Table 7-1.

Acute Clinical Indications

Since the majority of congenital malformations occur without history and the majority are not associated with a chromosomal or a mendelian basis, most are undetected prior to birth. Many malformations, however, produce clinical abnormalities during prenatal care and thereby identify candidates for ultrasonic evaluation and prenatal diagnosis. Abnormalities of uterine

Table 7-1. General Indications for Prenatal Diagnosis

1. Previous birth of a child with an inheritable disease or malformation for which techniques exist that allow prenatal diagnosis.
2. A family history of an inheritable disease that strongly suggests an increased risk of the birth of a child with that disease.
3. Maternal age over 35 years at the birth of the child. Paternal age over 55 years at the birth of the child.
4. Elevated maternal serum α-fetoprotein.
5. Established carrier status for a disease for which techniques exist that allow prenatal diagnosis.
6. Immediate clinical indications for sonography such as abnormal uterine size or fetal cardiac arrhythmia.

fundal growth and fetal heart rate are notable examples of acute clinical indications for prenatal diagnosis, usually by ultrasound.

Fundal Height Discrepancies

The uterine height, measured in centimeters from pubic symphysis to the top of the fundus, approximates the gestational age in weeks between weeks 20 and 35 (Fig 7-1). This clinical measure is a reflection of fetal mass and amniotic fluid, as well as uterus and placenta. A significant abnormality of any of these might alter the normal fundal height. Whenever fundal height in centimeters exceeds gestational age in weeks by 3 cm, or falls 4 cm short, referral for ultrasound examination is indicated.

The sonographic examination of a patient with a size/dates discrepancy focuses on confirmation of gestational age, assessment of amniotic fluid volume, and evaluation of uterine anomalies.

Abnormalities of Amniotic Fluid Volume

When a fundal height discrepancy is the result of an abnormality of amniotic fluid, either an excess or a deficiency, a careful fetal anatomical examination is indicated. Amniotic fluid is a physiological extension of the fetus. Severe oligohydramnios (Fig 7-2) early in gestation often results from blockage, agenesis, or dysplasia of the fetal urinary tract. Ruptured mem-

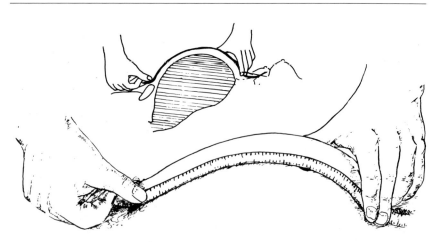

Fig 7-1. Fundal height. Method for measuring fundal height from the top of the pubic symphysis to the top of a uterine fundus using a flexible centimeter tape.

Fetal limbs
Fetal spine
Fetal body
Rib
Placenta

B

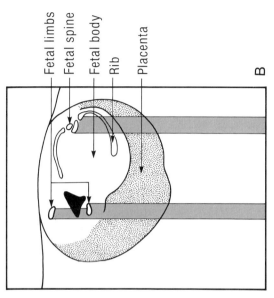

Fig 7-2. Oligohydramnios. (*A*) This transverse uterine scan of a pregnancy at approximately 19 weeks' gestation demonstrates the absence of amniotic fluid. (*B*) Diagram emphasizes the important anatomical features shown in the sonogram.

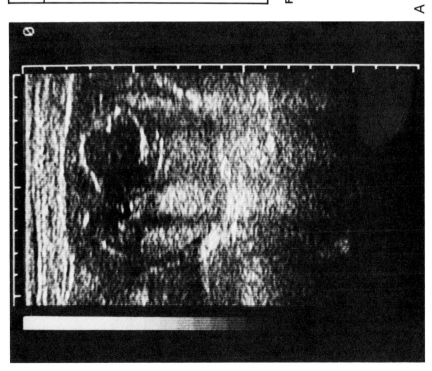

A

branes must also be ruled out. Neonatal salvage in cases of severe, early oligohydramnios is rare.

Hydramnios (formerly polyhydramnios) can be associated with diabetes mellitus, erythroblastosis fetalis, major malformations, or idiopathic causes (Fig 7-3). If diabetes and blood group incompatibilities are excluded by clinical evaluation, fetal malformations are found in almost half of the remaining cases.

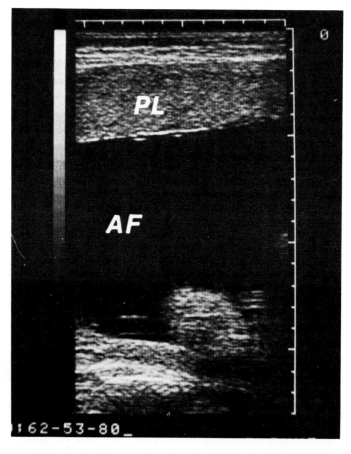

Fig 7-3. Hydramnios. When the uterus is excessively large for dates, and the excess size is found to be due to amniotic fluid (AF), the sonographic appearance will be similar to that shown in this sonogram. (PL, placenta)

Fetal malformations associated with hydramnios include obstructive lesions of the proximal bowel such as esophageal or duodenal atresia and nonintestinal mass lesions of the fetal abdomen that produce obstruction from compression and distortion. Abnormalities of the fetal chest such as congenital hydrothorax, diaphragmatic hernia, or severe cardiomegaly are associated with hydramnios presumably through increased intrathoracic pressure or direct esophageal compression. Myotonic dystrophy in the fetus is strongly associated with hydramnios, probably because of decreased esophageal tone. As will be seen in Chapter 9, many of these lesions present a characteristic sonographic image and are detectable prenatally.

Fetal Cardiac Arrhythmias

A fetal arrhythmia may be a clue to the presence of an intracardiac malformation. A persistent fetal bradyarrhythmia can be the result of complete heart block associated with maternal collagen vascular disease or result from fetal cardiac structural abnormalities that prevent normal atrioventricular conduction. An endocardial cushion defect is such an example. Fetal M-mode echocardiography (M = motion) allows confirmation of normal ventricular and atrial architecture and often allows differential assessment of the synchrony of atrial and ventricular activity (Fig 7-4). This can allow identification of the site of conduction block.

Maternal Serum α-Fetoprotein

α-Fetoprotein (AFP) is a product of the fetal liver and is similar to albumin. It is a constituent of fetal blood that is excreted into amniotic fluid, and small amounts are found in maternal serum during early pregnancy. Maternal serum levels of AFP (MSAFP) are elevated in cases of fetomaternal hemorrhage and a variety of fetal malformations. Open neural tube defects result in elevated levels of AFP in amniotic fluid and secondarily in maternal serum. Fetal gastroschisis and omphalocele also lead to increased amniotic fluid AFP and MSAFP levels. Fetal renal agenesis, complete urinary obstruction, and certain renal dysplasias also result in increased MSAFP.

MSAFP may be assayed by immunological methods, and such testing is available in some areas on a routine basis as a screen for malformations. The diagnostic threshold for designating a level as elevated differs from laboratory to laboratory and varies with race, maternal weight, and gestational age. An apparent elevation might be the result of incorrect gestational dates, unsuspected fetal death, twins, fetal malformations mentioned previously, or unknown causes. An elevation of MSAFP is another clinical

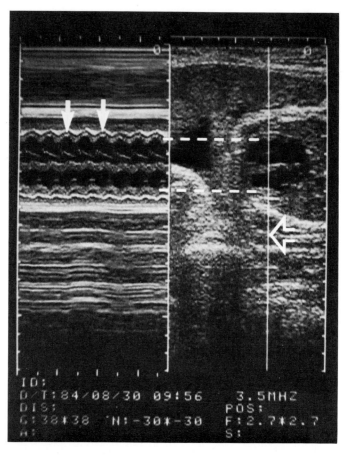

Fig 7-4. Normal fetal echocardiogram. The image on the left represents the moving echos detected along the scan line indicated by the open arrow. The dashed lines indicate the
relationship between the two-dimensional anatomy of the lateral ventricular walls and the moving structures in the M-
mode scan. The two solid arrows indicate the movement of
the lateral wall of the right ventricle. In this echocardiogram
the contractions of both ventricles may be seen to be synchronous and regular.

indication for sonographic evaluation to assess gestational age and fetal viability and number, and if simple explanation is not found, a careful fetal morphologic examination should be performed by operators experienced at prenatal sonographic diagnosis. Recently, low MSAFP has been related to fetal cytogenetic abnormalities and may indicate the need for evaluation.

PRENATAL DIAGNOSIS: ULTRASOUND

Ultrasound has demonstrated the ability to detect fetal malformations that cause the distortion or distention of fetal organs. Fluid accumulates within the obstructed system and allows visualization of the defective organ. The lateral ventricles of the brain in hydrocephalus, the distended bladder obstructed by urethral valves, and the cystic kidney with ureteropelvic junction obstruction are examples. The stomach becomes distended secondary to outlet obstruction in the form of duodenal atresia, annular pancreas, or intraluminal webs. Specific cardiac chambers may become distended secondary to valvular stenosis or atresia.

It is the echo contrast of the fluid and adjacent soft tissue that allows visualization of these lesions. Amniotic fluid outside the fetus is also important to the diagnosis of surface lesions of the fetus, such as clefting of the face or spina bifida. The soft tissue anatomy is clear only when contrasted to surrounding fluid. In the absence of amniotic fluid, such as in the case of renal agenesis, image quality is poor and precise diagnosis is difficult. Fluid, then, because of its homogeneity and absence of echos, is the critical contrast medium of the ultrasonographer. Fluid of some type, or absence of it, is critical to the majority of successful prenatal diagnoses made with ultrasound.

Specific indications for the use of ultrasound in prenatal diagnosis include the following:

- Assignment or confirmation of gestational age to allow accurate interpretation of other maternal or fetal serum or amniotic fluid tests
- Prior to amniocentesis for date confirmation, placental and fetal localization, and fetal anatomical examination
- Guidance of invasive diagnostic techniques such as amniocentesis, fetoscopy, or fetal intervention
- Visual diagnosis of fetal morphologic malformations in those patients believed to be at risk for a visible lesion either on historical or clinical grounds

SUGGESTED READINGS

Canty TG, Leopold GR, Wolf DA: Maternal ultrasonography for the antenatal diagnosis of surgically significant neonatal anomalies. *Ann Surg* 194:353–365, 1981.

Chamberlain PF, Manning FA, Morrison I, et al: Ultrasound evaluation of amniotic fluid volume: I. The relationship of marginal and decreased amniotic fluid volumes to perinatal outcome. *Am J Obstet Gynecol* 150:245–249, 1984.

Hill LM, Breckle R, Gehrking WC: Prenatal detection of congenital malformations by ultrasonography: Mayo Clinic experience. *Am J Obstet Gynecol* 151:44–50, 1985.

Jacoby HE, Charles D: Clinical conditions associated with hydramnios. *Am J Obstet Gynecol* 94:910–919, 1966.

Mercer LJ, Brown LG, Petres RE, et al: A survey of pregnancies complicated by decreased amniotic fluid. *Am J Obstet Gynecol* 149:355–361, 1984.

Nicolini U, Ferrazzi E, Kustermann A, et al: Effectiveness of routine ultrasound in screening congenital defects *J Perinatol Med* 10:125–129, 1982.

Skovbo P, Smith-Jensen S: Ultrasonic scanning and fetography at polyhydramnios. *Acta Obstet Gynecol Scand* 60:51–54, 1981.

Verma U, Weiss RR, Almonte R, et al: Early prenatal diagnosis of soft tissue malformations. *Obstet Gynecol* 53:660–663, 1979.

Wong WS, Filly RA: Polyhydramnios associated with fetal limb abnormalities. *AJR* 140:1001–1003, 1983.

Zamah NM, Gillieson MS, Walters JH, et al: Sonographic detection of polyhydramnios: A five-year experience. *Am J Obstet Gynecol* 143:523–527, 1982.

Chapter 8

Prenatal Sonographic Appearance of Congenital Malformations

CRANIOSPINAL MALFORMATIONS

Anencephaly, encephalocele, and lumbosacral spina bifida (spinal dysraphia) are neural tube defects that may be diagnosed with ultrasound. Cervical cystic hygroma and nuchal teratomas are also malformations of this anatomical region that are potentially detectable with ultrasound. Ninety-five percent of these anomalies occur in families with no previous history of such a defect.

In order to provide maximum diagnostic sensitivity to these disorders, a careful assessment of the skull, intracranial anatomy, and spinal column should be included in all obstetrical ultrasound examinations.

Anencephaly

Half of all neural tube defects (failure of closure of the primitive neural tube in the early embryo) involve absence of the cranial vault. Orbits and face are formed, and often irregular soft tissue structures are seen, suggesting imperfect attempts to form brain tissue (Fig 8-1). An association between anencephaly and breech presentation emphasizes the need for sonographic evaluation of patients with malpresentation to rule out major malformations, including anencephaly. Anencephaly is uniformly fatal, although exceptional cases might survive several months.

The fetal cranium should be consistently seen with ultrasound by 14 weeks' gestation. At any gestational age, the cranium is usually the easiest fetal organ to image and recognize. If a cranium is not easily found, the spine may be located and the transducer aligned with it and then moved cranially. Failure to locate the cranial vault despite careful study by 14 weeks' gestation with contemporary realtime equipment is diagnostic of anencephaly. Occasionally, deep pelvic engagement of the fetal cranium

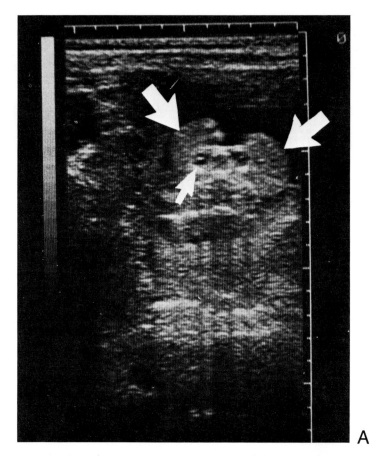

A

Fig 8-1. Anencephaly. (*A*) Frontal view of the face of an anencephalic
fetus. The small arrow indicates one orbit; the larger arrows
indicate soft tissue masses originating from the base of the
skull, which are frequently observed in anencephaly. (*B*) Sagittal
view of an anencephalic fetus. The solid triangle illustrates
one orbit. No cranium is seen above this level.

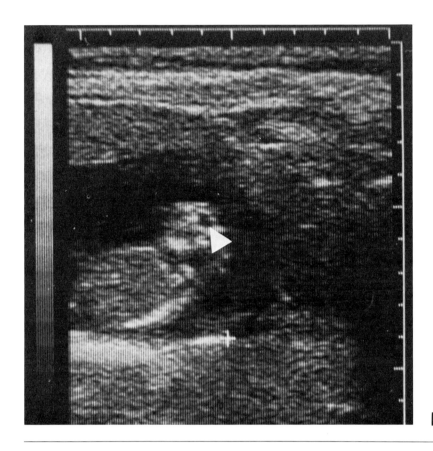

B

might mimic anencephaly, and in those cases in which the fetal cervical spine extends over the pelvic brim with poor clarity of deeper anatomy, a simultaneous pelvic examination should be performed to elevate the presenting part of the fetus out of the pelvis and allow more complete visualization.

Spina Bifida

The fetal spine should be examined both longitudinally and transversely (Fig 8-2). Careful study by an experienced examiner can result in the diagnosis of up to 80% of spinal defects. In the case of a dysraphic (bifid) lesion, the neural canal fails to close, leading to open communication of the subarachnoid space with the amniotic cavity or herniation of the intact meninges and formation of a meningocele. In such cases, longitudinal imaging should be performed of the posterolateral spinal echocenters (plane

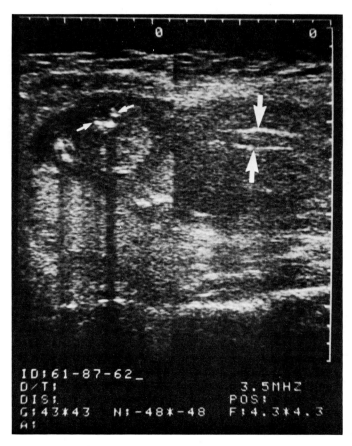

A

Fig 8-2. Spina bifida. (*A* and *B*) In both of these views of a fetus with spina bifida, the right-hand scan is a longitudinal view of the posterolateral spinal elements and demonstrates a widening or separation of these elements (arrows). Compare these views to the normal fetal appearance illustrated in Figure 3-6. The left-hand view in both of these scans is a transverse scan of the same spine at the level of the marker on the right. These transverse views, which also show a separation of the posterolateral echogenic elements of the spine and of open appearance posteriorly, may be compared with normal views in Figure 3-5*A*.

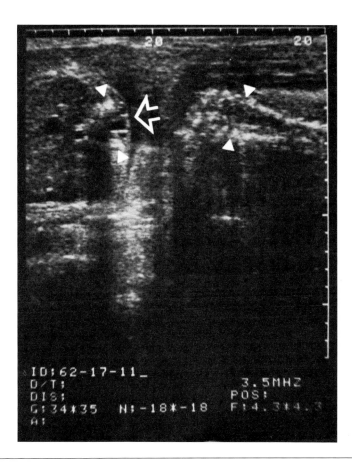

B

A of Fig 3-5B) and will demonstrate a separation of these centers in the area of the defect (Fig 8-3). Serial transverse scanning should show a wide separation of the posterolateral echocenters in the region of the defect, often with open communication posteriorly. Rare cases will show complete failure of neural tube closure, called craniospinal rachischisis (Fig 8-4). A lipomyelomeningocele is a rare intraspinal lipomatous tumor associated with occult spina bifida that appears as an echogenic soft tissue mass dorsal to a dysraphic spinal lesion (Fig 8-5).

Encephalocele

Another possible result of failure of the rostral neuropore to close is an encephalocele. This is a cystic lesion arising from the occipital midline of

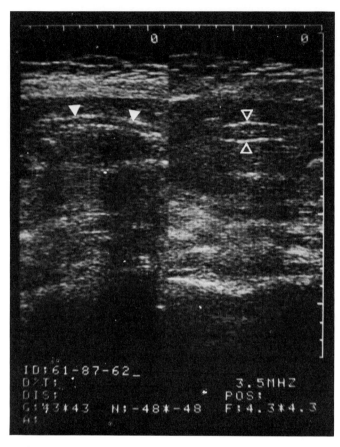

ID:61-87-62_
D.T:
DIS:
G:43+43   N:-48*-48   F:4.3*4.3
A:
3.5MHZ
POS:

A

Fig 8-3. Spina bifida. (A) Longitudinal views of the same fetal spine.
The view on the right (open triangles) corresponds to the scan
plane illustrated by plane A in Figure 3-5B. The left-hand scan
is of the same fetal spine (solid triangles) corresponding to
plane B in Figure 3-5B and illustrates that this is not as sensitive a view. (B) The widening of these posterolateral elements
indicates spina bifida, which was confirmed at examination of
the abortus.

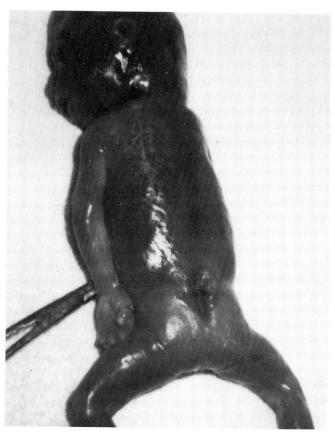

B

the fetal cranium (Fig 8-6). Encephaloceles are essentially cranial meningoceles and may contain neural tissue or be filled only with fluid. Anechoic, discretely demarcated, nonseptate masses arising from the occipital area are most likely encephaloceles. They may be large or small and may be associated with other abnormalities such as hydrocephalus.

Hydrocephalus

Hydrocephalus may be an isolated finding associated with aqueductal stenosis or may accompany spina bifida. Whenever hydrocephalus is diagnosed, a careful examination of the fetal spine should follow. Hydrocephalus is a dilatation of the ventricular system of the brain usually secondary to outflow obstruction. Diagnosis is based on the observation of lateral ventric-

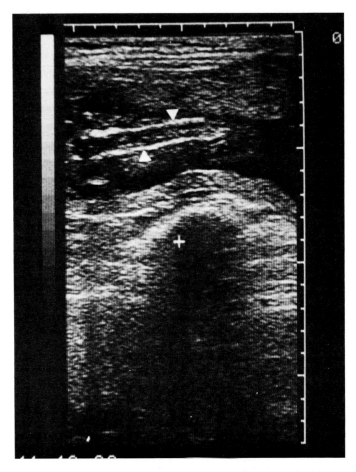

Fig 8-4. Craniospinal rachischisis. This longitudinal view of the posterolateral elements of a fetal spine demonstrates wide separation of the entire length of the fetal spine (solid triangles). This fetus demonstrated completely open neural tube with anencephaly. The two rows of echo centers appear parallel.

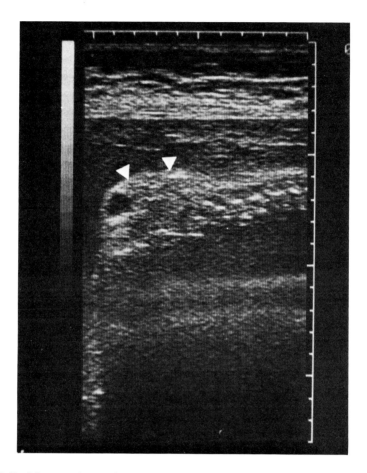

Fig 8-5. Lipomyelomeningocele. The solid triangles indicate an echogenic soft tissue mass dorsal to a spinal defect. This is the ultrasonic appearance of a lipoma originating within the neural canal. *Source:* Adapted with permission from *Obstetrics and Gynecology* (1986), Copyright © 1986, Elsevier Science Publishing Company, Inc.

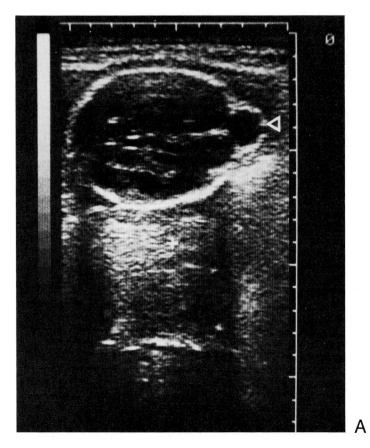

A

Fig 8-6. Encephalocele. Encephaloceles originate from the occipito-frontal midline and may be small (*A*) or large (*B*). They may or may not contain neural tissue and have a variable prognosis.

ular dilatation (Fig 8-7). This dilatation may be seen either at the anterior horns or in the area of the choroid plexes (Fig 8-8). The anterior horns may be seen and measured as early as 15 weeks' gestation. It is usually necessary to align the brain midline precisely perpendicular to the direction of propagation of the sound beam since the marginal membranes of the ventricles are thin and will not be seen if off axis. Both ventricles should be seen before measurement to ensure proper alignment. These spaces may then be measured with calipers.

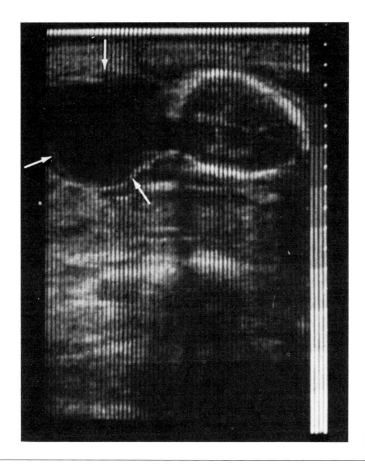

B

In cases in which isolated hydrocephalus is diagnosed, cortical mantle thickness may be serially measured and progression of cortical atrophy assessed (Fig 8-9). Fetal therapy of isolated symmetrical hydrocephalus in which progression is documented and other malformations are excluded might be considered in some perinatal centers. Placement of an indwelling ventriculoamniotic catheter can produce decompression of the ventricular system and reduce dilatation, but long-term benefits are unproven.

Hydrocephalus can also be associated with intracranial lesions such as porencephalic cysts (Fig 8-10) and cystic malformations of the posterior fossa (Fig 8-11), and it can be confused with unilobar holoprosencephaly (Fig 8-12). Neurobehavioral prognosis in cases of porencephaly and with

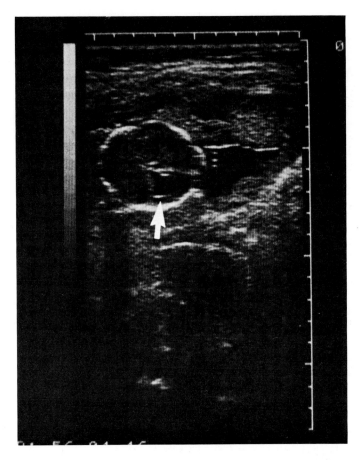

Fig 8-7. Early hydrocephalus. The frontal horn of the lateral ventricle of this 18-week fetus is dilated relative to the hemisphere (arrow). Compare this with the normal frontal horn illustrated in Figure 3-2.

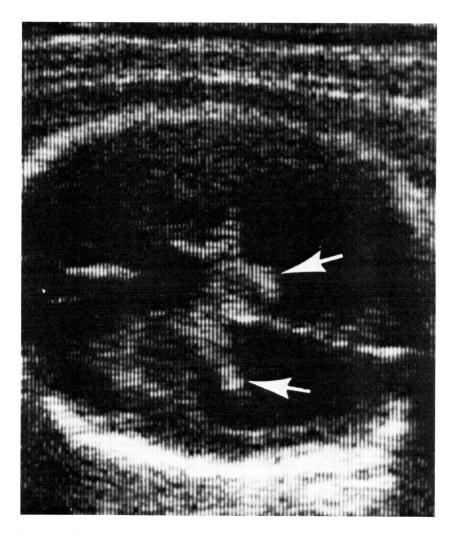

Fig 8-8. Choroid plexes in hydrocephalus: In the case of ventriculomegaly, choroid plexes normally droop unsupported within the posterolateral ventricle (arrows).

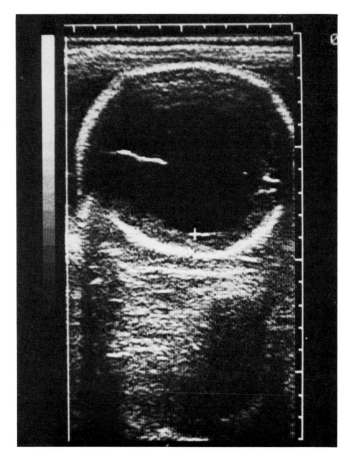

Fig 8-9. Cortical mantle. In this case of severe ventriculomegaly, measurement of the cortical mantle may be the most practical method of assessing progression in ventricular dilatation.

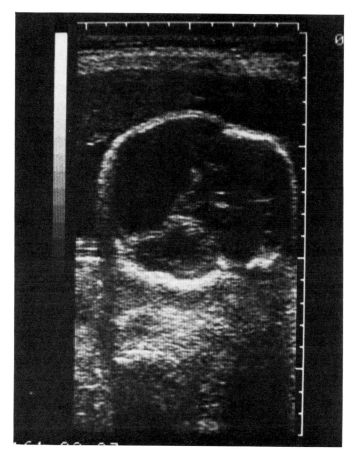

Fig 8-10. Porencephalic cysts. The irregular asymmetrical anechoic (black) cystic area in the upper posterior area of this occipito-frontal scan of a fetal cranium is typical of a porencephalic cyst. These may or may not be associated with hydrocephalus.

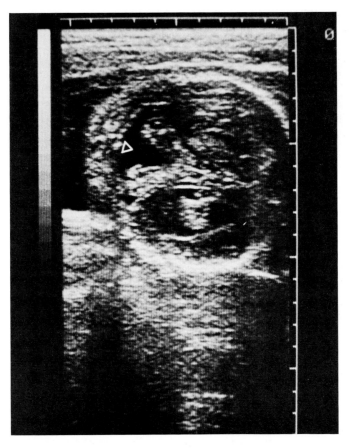

A

Fig 8-11. Dandy-Walker cysts. (*A*) Review the anatomy of the posterior fossa illustrated in Figure 3-3 and compare it with this view. The open triangle sits in the cisterna magna and is pointed toward a cleft between the cerebellar hemispheres, which is not normal. (*B*) Progression in the cystic dilatation of the fourth ventricle leads to complete cystic replacement of the posterior fossa (pf). The arrow indicates a fetal orbit.

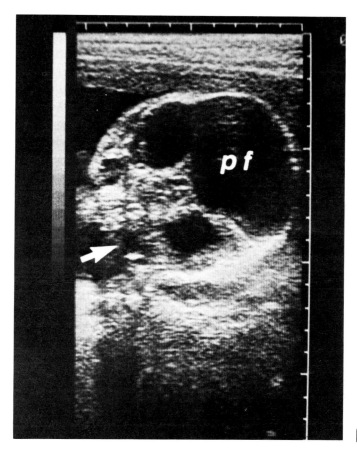

B

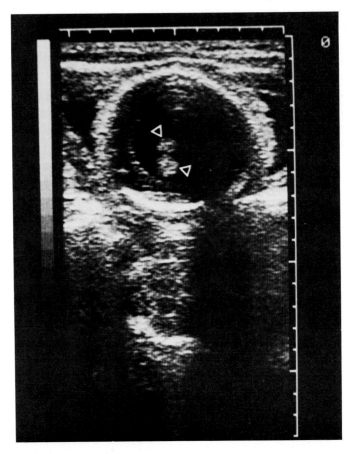

Fig 8-12. Holoprosencephaly. The open triangles indicate the choroid plexes within a single dilated central ventricle, which is a typical appearance of holoprosencephaly.

Dandy-Walker malformation is significantly worse than with isolated symmetrical hydrocephalus.

Cystic Hygroma

Congenital lymphangiectasia may produce anechoic masses in various locations. Most often seen in the area of the dorsal cervical spine (Fig 8-13), these anechoic masses are sharply outlined, are usually covered by skin, and show internal septa that represent the outlines of the dilated lymph channels of which they are composed. Cystic hygroma is often associated with generalized fetal hydrops and with 45X karyotype, and a fetus found to have such a lesion has a uniformly poor prognosis.

Teratomas of the Spine and Neck

Teratomas are congenital tumors that can arise in any part of the fetus. They are usually solid and complex, with disorganized structure and areas of calcification within them (Fig 8-14). Teratomas may be intracranial or arise from the lips, neck, or sacrum. They can appear totally cystic or solid, but most often they present a mixed pattern. Sacrococcygeal teratomas arise from the most caudal end of the fetal spine and may achieve large proportions (Fig 8-15). These lesions are usually skin covered. Neonatal excision and repair is often successful.

THORACOABDOMINAL MALFORMATIONS

Intracardiac defects, pleural effusions, chest wall defects, diaphragmatic hernia, ventral wall defects of the abdomen, obstructive lesions of the proximal and distal gut, and meconium peritonitis are all potentially detectable in the fetus with ultrasound.

Cardiac Defects

The fetal heart can be seen as early as 8 weeks' gestation, and clear anatomy of the four chambers may be demonstrated by 16 to 17 weeks' gestation. In the normal heart, the ventricles are of roughly equal size and synchronous contractility. Significant asymmetry or asynchrony suggests malformation. Aortic valvular atresia leads to a hypoactive left ventricle with thickening of the myocardium (Fig 8-16). Dilatation of the left atrium is associated with hydramnios, probably through pressure on the esophagus. An endocardial cushion defect results in dramatic visual disruption of the

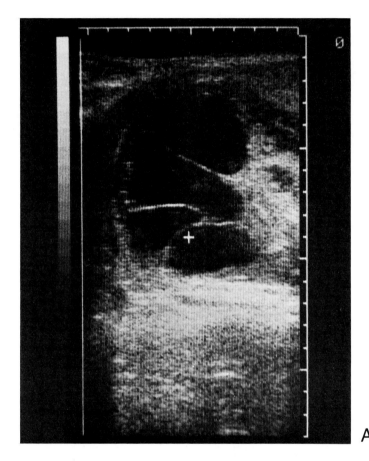

A

Fig 8-13. Cystic hygroma. (*A*) Sonogram of the multiloculated posterior cervical neck mass that is typical of a cystic hygroma. (*B*) Cystic hygroma represents obstruction of subcutaneous lymphatic channels.

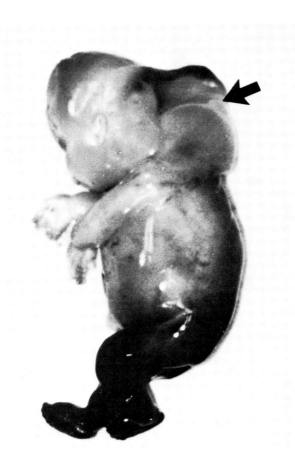

B

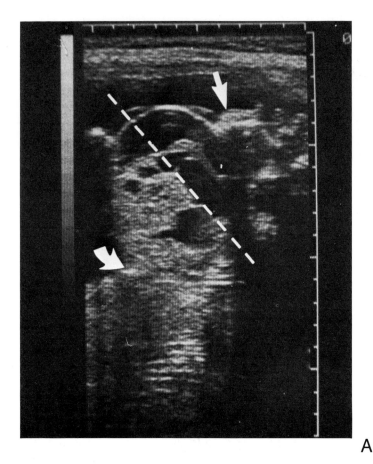

A

Fig 8-14. Nuchal teratoma. (*A*) Longitudinal midline scan extending
from the fetal chin (straight arrow) through the teratoma to
the top of the fetal chest (curved arrow). A teratoma fills the
anterior neck and is extending the fetal head dorsally. The
teratoma may be seen to contain both cystic (black) and
solid areas. (*B*) Transverse scan of this neck mass at the
level indicated by the dashed line. The solid (s) and cystic (c)
areas are clearly seen. This is the typical disorganized anatomy of a teratoma.

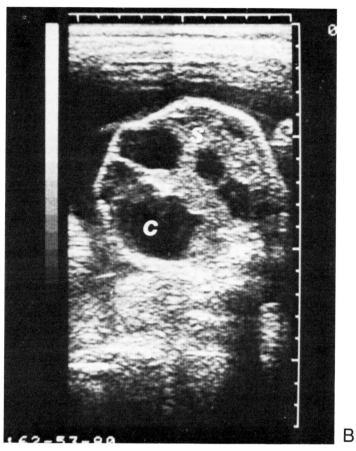

B

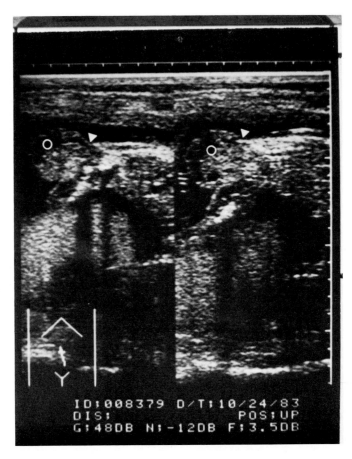

Fig 8-15. Sacrococcygeal teratoma. The solid triangles in these scans indicate the approximate area of the sacrum. To the left of the solid triangle is a circular, echogenic, soft tissue mass (circles) that is a sacrococcygeal teratoma. These may also be purely cystic.

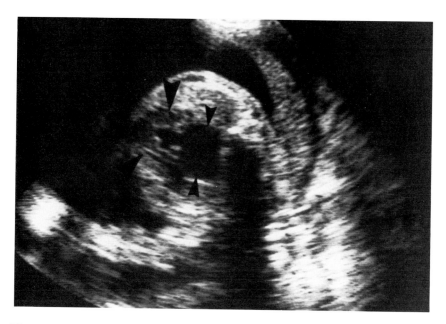

Fig 8-16. Aortic valvular atresia. Aortic valvular atresia results in a thick-walled left ventricle (large arrowhead) and a dilated thin-walled left atrium (small arrowheads). The contractile activity of this left ventricle will be seen diminished.

central anatomy of the heart often also causing atrial enlargement (Fig 8-17). A single atrium–single ventricle complex (Fig 8-18) is often but not always fatal and may be clinically selected for ultrasound examination because of persistent fetal bradycardia.

Ventral chest wall defects are relatively rare and include a family of lesions from simple sternal clefts to ectopia cordis (Fig 8-19). Sternal clefting with diaphragmatic dysplasia can lead to cardiac displacement, which ought to be visible with ultrasound.

In the prenatal management of a fetal cardiac malformation, serial sonography can be helpful in assessing the impact of the defect on cardiac hemodynamics. Ascites, effusions, and widespread edema are indications of fetal venous hypertension often associated with pump failure. Consideration might be given to delivery if hydrops develops, or to digitalis therapy if the pregnancy is remote from term.

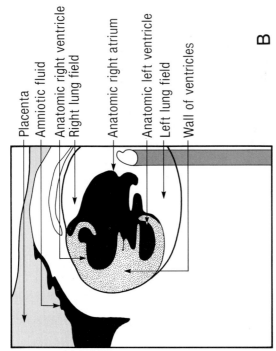

Placenta
Amniotic fluid
Anatomic right ventricle
Right lung field
Anatomic right atrium
Anatomic left ventricle
Left lung field
Wall of ventricles

B

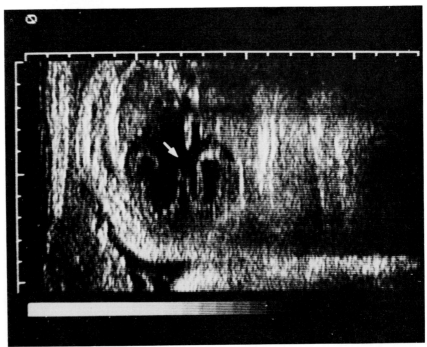

A

Fig 8-17. Endocardial cushion defect. (A) Sonogram of an enlarged fetal heart with confluence of the ventricles and the right atrium. Open passage between the right atrium and both ventricles (arrow) is consistent with the diagnosis of an endocardial cushion defect. (B) Major anatomical features are illustrated. This fetus presented with persistent bradycardia and polyhydramnios.

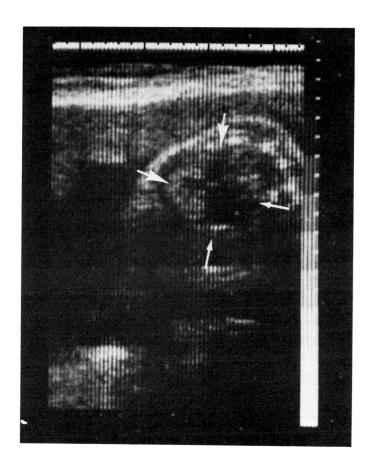

Fig 8-18. Single atrium/ventricle. This fetus was found to demonstrate persistent bradycardia and on scan was seen to have a single irregular ventricle (large arrows) and a single large atrium (small arrows). Compare this view with the normal heart illustrated in Figure 3-8*A*.

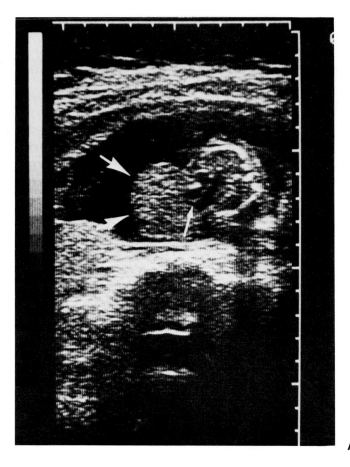

A

Fig 8-19. Combined thoracoabdominal defect. (*A*) Sonogram of the upper fetal abdomen shows an omphalocele (large arrows) originating from the anterior fetus. The ventricles of the heart (small arrow) are seen extended from the fetal chest into the upper portion of the omphalocele. (*B*) Abortus confirms the sonographic findings. *Source:* Adapted with permission from *Prenatal Diagnosis* (1984;4), Copyright © 1984, John Wiley & Sons Ltd.

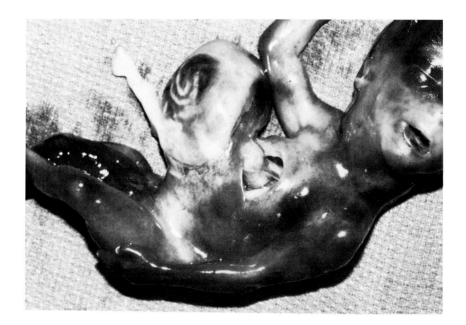

B

Echocardiography

The study of the rhythm and excursion of echos located along a single scan line as a function of time is called time motion study (or T-M mode or simply M-mode). Such studies are useful for assessing contractility, by measuring the rate of movement of cardiac structures including valves. More commonly, the differential evaluation of atrial and ventricular synchrony can allow the diagnosis of fetal arrhythmias (Fig 8-20).

Hydrothorax

Congenital pleural effusions are visible with ultrasound. Pleural effusions produce an anechoic (black) layer surrounding the lungs (Fig 8-21). The

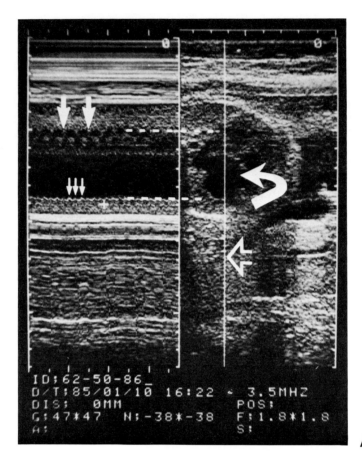

A

Fig 8-20. Fetal arrhythmias. (A) Echocardiogram performed on a fetus with atrial flutter and a 2:1 atrioventricular block. The small arrows on the left indicate atrial wall activity at twice the rate of ventricular response indicated by the large arrows. The curved arrow on the right indicates the enlarged right atrium. Open arrow indicates M-mode beam location. (B) Echocardiogram of a fetus with an irregular heart beat. The arrows indicate ventricular activity and the third arrow from the left indicates a premature ventricular contraction with a compen-

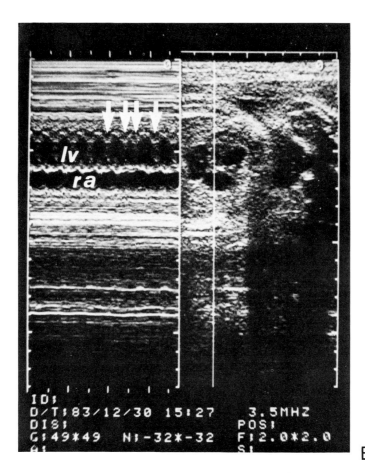

B

satory pause. lv = blood in left ventricle; ra = blood in right atrium. (*C*) Complete heart block. The echos on the left of this echocardiogram originate along the line indicated by the large solid arrow. The large arrows on the left indicate ventricular activity, and the small arrows indicate atrial activity. (*D*) Echocardiogram of a fetus with bigeminal rhythm. The arrows indicate ventricular activity in a paired bigeminy-type rhythm.

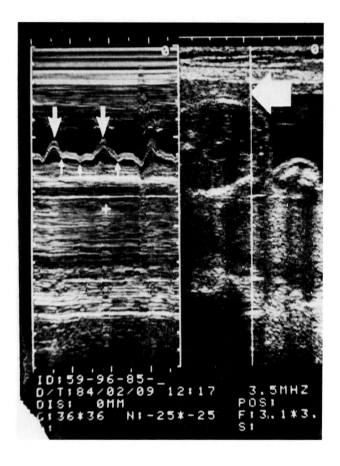

C

Fig 8-20. Continued.

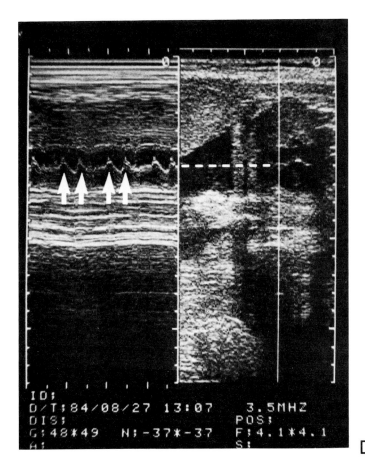

D

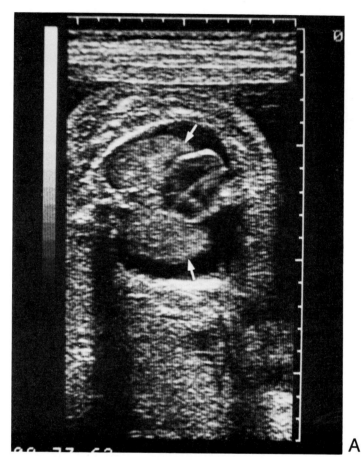

Fig 8-21. Fetal hydrothorax. (A) Transverse fetal chest illustrating hydrothorax. The pleural fluid (black) clearly outlines the lungs (arrows) and the heart. (B) Longitudinal scan of the same fetus with the solid triangles indicating the fetal lungs projecting into the pleural fluid (black). *Source:* Adapted with permission from *Obstetrics and Gynecology* (1986), Copyright © 1986, Elsevier Science Publishing Company, Inc.

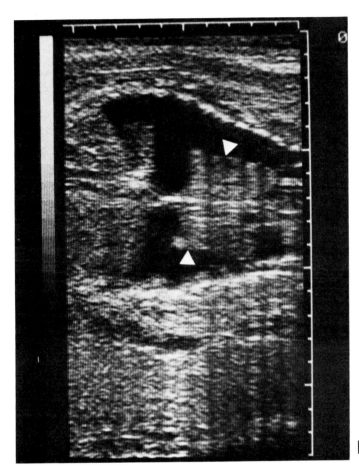

B

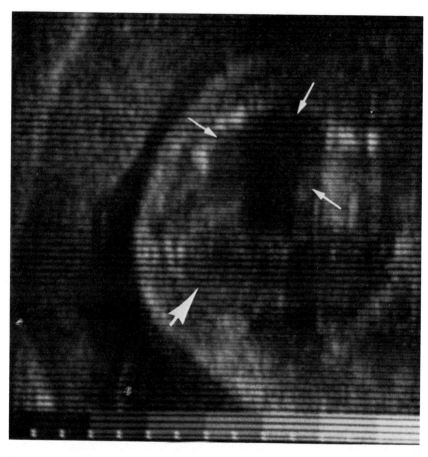

Fig 8-22. Diaphragmatic hernia. This transverse scan of the fetal chest illustrates cardiac activity (large arrow) displaced to the right side by a large cystic mass (small arrows) consistent with the diagnosis of herniated stomach and diaphragmatic hernia.

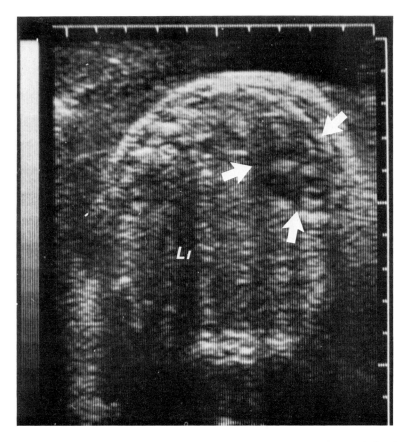

Fig 8-23. Right diaphragmatic hernia. This transverse scan of the fetal chest illustrates dramatic left displacement of the fetal heart (arrows) and migration of the liver (Li) into the right chest.

effusions may grow to large proportions and if asymmetrical may even displace the mediastinal structures. Effusions may be associated with generalized fetal hydrops or be isolated lesions.

Diaphragmatic Hernia

The lung fields on either side of the heart should be homogeneous and free of anechoic (black) or cystic areas. The heart and mediastinum should be just slightly to the left of center. Ninety percent of diaphragmatic hernias occur on the left side of the chest and appear as cystic masses to the left of the heart, often with displacement of the heart to the right (Fig 8-22). If the

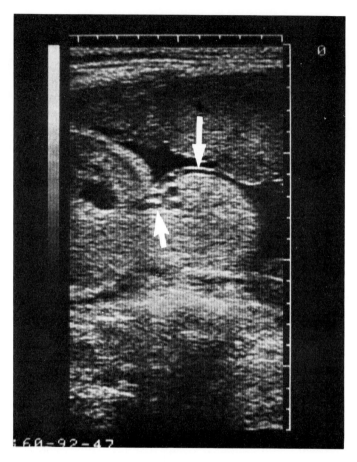

Fig 8-24. Omphalocele. Omphalocele arises from the lower anterior midline of the fetal abdomen and comprises a soft tissue mass surrounded by a thin membrane (long arrow). The umbilical vessels are seen here to pass from the omphalocele into the fetal abdomen (small arrow).

defect is on the right, the liver could be displaced upward into the chest and the heart would be moved to the left (Fig 8-23). Hydramnios is a common clinical correlate to diaphragmatic hernias of both sides.

Ventral Abdominal Wall Defects

Ventral wall defects such as gastroschisis and omphalocele involve a disruption of the integrity of the anterior abdominal wall. The omphalocele is a failure of the embryonic gut to return to the abdominal cavity during early embryogenesis. Abdominal viscera remain in the proximal umbilical cord. The size varies, but the extrophied gut or liver is typically covered by a peritoneal-like membrane (Fig 8-24). Sonographic detection of even the smallest omphalocele is based on careful serial transverse scanning of the fetal abdomen at the umbilicus. Gastroschisis also involves extrophied abdominal organs, but from a site apart from the umbilicus (Fig 8-25). Gastroschisis is due probably to an embryonic vascular accident. The eviscerated organs in this case are not covered by any membrane. Since amniotic fluid induces an inflammatory reaction in the serosal surface of the intestines, the extrophied gut often appears intensely echogenic and thick walled. Hydramnios is often a clinical association, as well as elevated levels of maternal serum α-fetoprotein.

Obstructed Stomach

Outlet obstruction of the fetal stomach results in both dilatation of the stomach and hydramnios. Often, cystic dilatation of the proximal duodenum is also seen (Fig 8-26). The obstruction may be on the basis of duodenal atresia or secondary to encroachment of an annular pancreas. Intraluminal duodenal webs are another possible cause of congenital stomach obstruction. Esophageal atresia, conversely, causes hydramnios with no stomach filling at all despite repeated examinations.

Bowel Perforation

Obstruction of the gut can lead to dilatation and perforation (Fig 8-27). Obstruction may be mechanical or functional. Meconium ileus may be seen with cystic fibrosis and can lead to perforation and peritonitis. The meconium peritonitis associated with bowel perforation produces an intense inflammatory response with calcifications in the late stage (Fig 8-28). Hydramnios is also a correlative finding. Hyperperistalsis may be seen near the area of perforation.

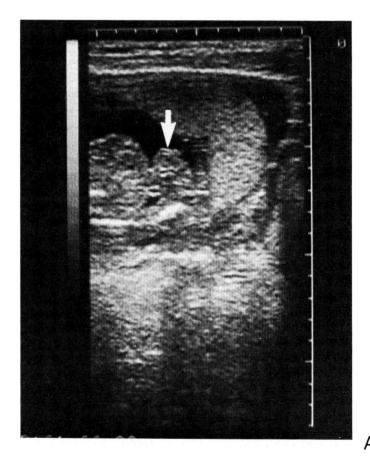

A

Fig 8-25. Gastroschisis. Gastroschisis appears to be a simple defect in the fetal ventral wall allowing escape of small bowel and other viscera into the amniotic cavity. (*A*) Defect in a 17-week fetus with herniated small bowel (arrow) free in the amniotic cavity. (*B*) Same fetus at 33 weeks' gestation. The loops of small bowel (large arrow) are more apparent, as is the echogenic thickening of the small bowel wall. The fetal abdominal wall (small arrows) is evident.

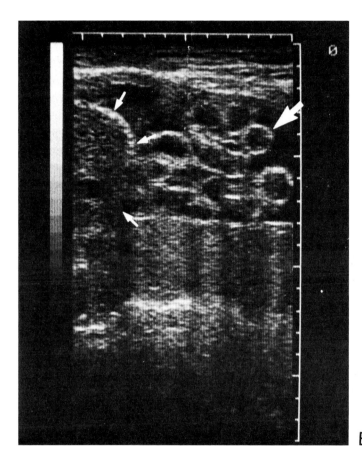

B

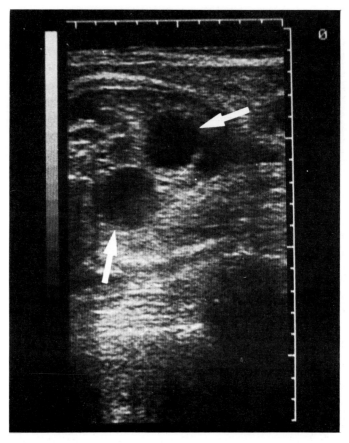

A

Fig 8-26. Fetal stomach obstruction. (*A*) Paired echolucent (black) masses of the upper abdomen (arrows) associated with duodenal atresia. (*B*) Obstruction associated with an annular pancreas (arrows) and not to duodenal atresia.

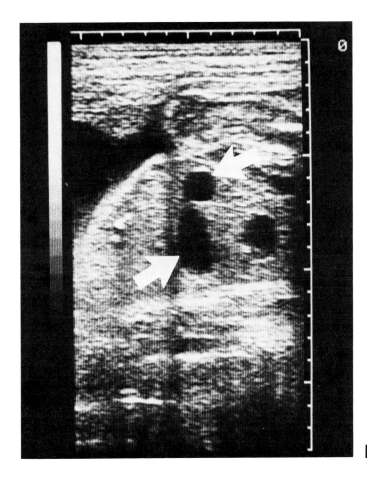

B

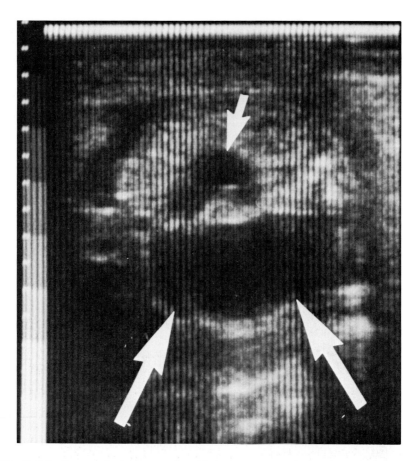

Fig 8-27. Congenital megacolon. This transverse lower fetal abdominal view demonstrates the large anechoic (black) mass associated with congenital fetal megacolon (arrows).

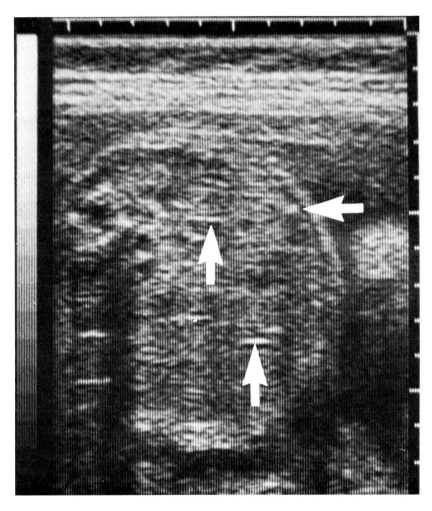

Fig 8-28. Meconium peritonitis. Rupture of fetal bowel causes meconium peritonitis and results in inflammation and calcification of areas within the fetal abdomen (arrows).

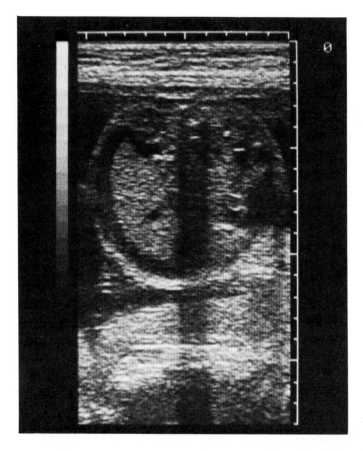

A

Fig 8-29. Ascites—hydrops. (*A* and *B*) Free peritoneal fluid appears as echolucent (black) material surrounding fetal organs. Ascites may (*B*) or may not (*A*) be associated with significant skin edema.

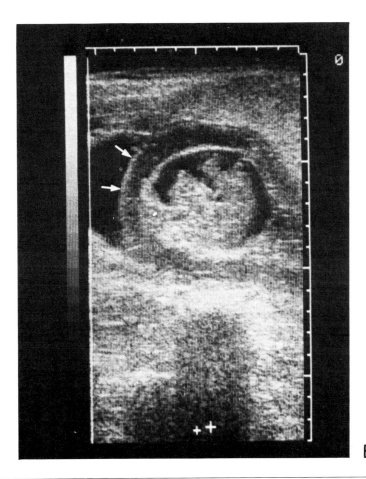

B

Ascites

Echo-spared areas outlining abdominal viscera may or may not be associated with other findings, such as generalized hydrops fetalis or even ruptured bowel or bladder (Fig 8-29).

URINARY TRACT ANOMALIES

The urinary tract is the site of origin of half of all congenital abdominal masses. Obstructive lesions predominate. Ureteropelvic junction obstruction is the most common obstructive lesion. Prenatal diagnosis can lead directly to neonatal treatment with organ salvage. Many of these would otherwise go undetected until later in childhood. Complete bilateral obstruction may or may not be associated with severe oligohydramnios, while unilateral obstruction is not. Unilateral obstruction can indirectly lead to hydramnios if a large mass results in proximal bowel compression or displacement.

Ureteropelvic Junction Obstruction

A large anechoic (black) paraspinal mass with distinct margins and a normal contralateral kidney is likely to be a ureteropelvic junction (UPJ) obstruction (Fig 8-30). The mass is typically symmetrical and free of internal structure. The visible mass may represent a perinephric urinoma associated with UPJ obstructions. Prenatal intervention is usually not warranted with these lesions because prompt neonatal treatment leads to salvage of a majority of kidneys.

Posterior Urethral Valves

Posterior urethral valves occur only in males and result in bladder outlet obstruction, usually with a greatly enlarged bladder (Fig 8-31) and bilateral hydronephrosis (Fig 8-32). Rupture of any segment of the urinary system results in often massive ascites (Fig 8-33). Oligohydramnios is an expected correlate of bladder outlet obstruction.

Cloacal Plate Anomalies

Failure of appropriate differentiation of the various derivatives of the cloacal plate results in a varied family of malformations that often demonstrate obstruction of both the bladder and bowel and often of communication between bladder, bowel, and even urachus (Fig 8-34). Such malformations usually occur in female phenotypes and result in severe oligohydramnios combined with a large fetal abdominal mass of irregular outline. The mass is usually larger than the simple obstructed bladder and of distinctly less symmetrical shape (Fig 8-35). Survival under any circumstances is rare, since pulmonary hypoplasia is usually present.

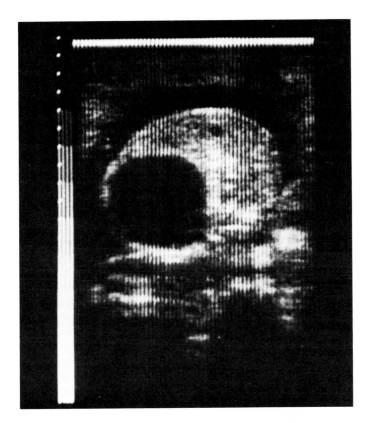

Fig 8-30. Fetal ureteropelvic junction obstruction. Transverse midabdominal view of a fetal trunk illustrating the large, discrete, anechoic (black) cystic mass associated with ureteropelvic junction obstruction.

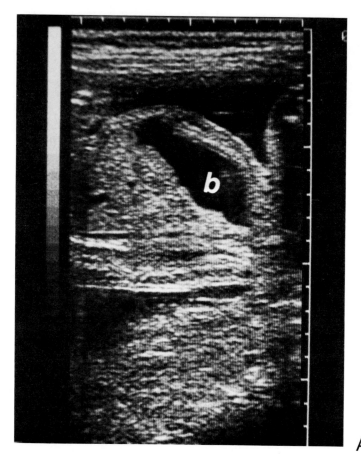

A

Fig 8-31. Fetal bladder obstruction. (*A*) Large obstructed fetal bladder (b). (*B*) Longitudinal view further illustrates the hydronephrotic kidneys (large arrows) as well as the dilated thick-walled fetal bladder (small arrow).

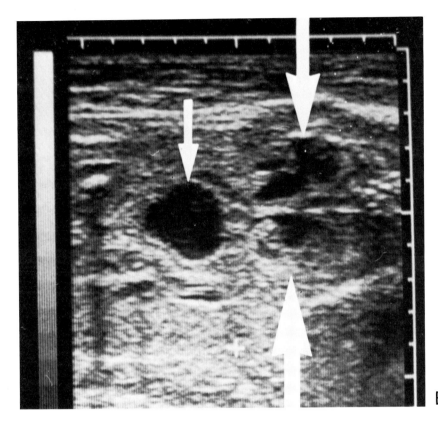

B

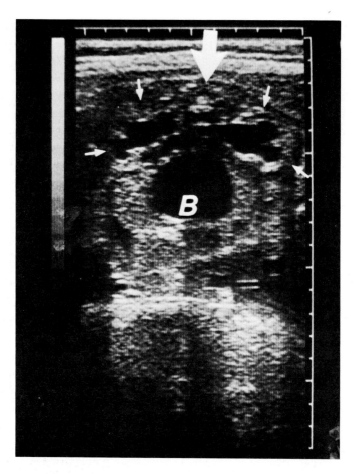

Fig 8-32. Fetal bladder obstruction. Transverse midabdominal view illustrates the dilated obstructed fetal bladder (B), as well as the bilateral hydronephrosis (small arrows). Large arrow indicates fetal spine.

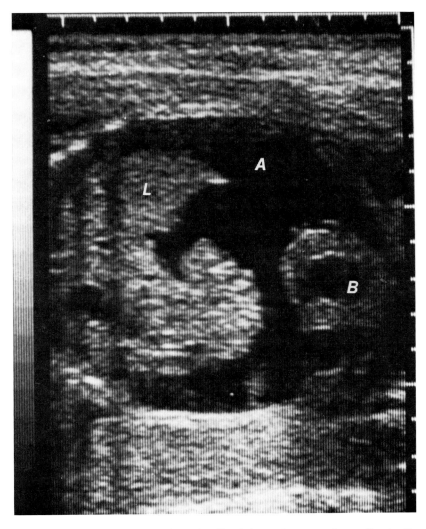

Fig 8-33. Urinary ascites. Longitudinal frontal scan plane illustrating the severe ascites associated with rupture of obstructed urinary tract. The liver (L) projects freely into the ascitic fluid (A). The thick-walled, partially contracted bladder (B) is easily seen.

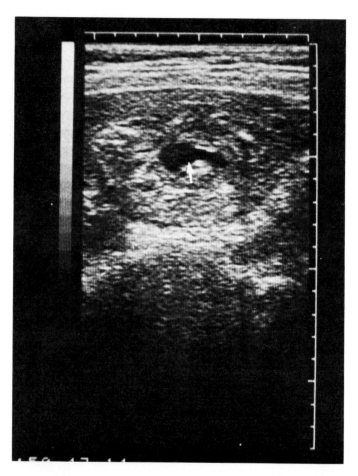

Fig 8-34. Cloacal plate malformation complex. Severe oligohydramnios combined with an irregular cystic mass (arrow) of the fetal abdomen strongly suggests the presence of cloacal plate anomaly complex rather than simple bladder obstruction.

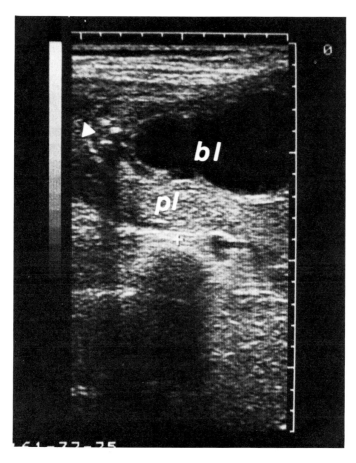

Fig 8-35. Bladder–bowel obstruction complex. This transverse abdominal scan of a fetus with severe oligohydramnios demonstrates a large, irregular cystic mass of the fetal abdomen that was found to comprise both bowel and bladder (bl). The solid triangle indicates the fetal spine casting an expected acoustical shadow. (pl, placental tissue.)

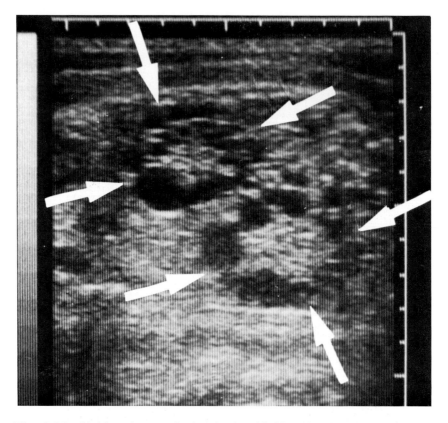

Fig 8-36. Multicystic renal dysplasia. Multicystic dysplasia demonstrates large macroscopic cystic masses (black) within the fetal kidneys. This transverse midabdominal scan demonstrates enlarged kidneys (arrows) with multiple macroscopic cysts.

Renal Dysplasia

Multicystic renal dysplasia is a congenital renal lesion presenting multiple macroscopic renal parenchymal cysts (Fig 8-36). The majority of cases are unilateral, and so normal amniotic fluid volumes are expected. When a normal contralateral kidney is present, survival is the rule.

Infantile polycystic renal dysplasia produces enlarged, hyperechoic kidneys and is usually bilateral (Fig 8-37). Multiple microscopic cysts of the

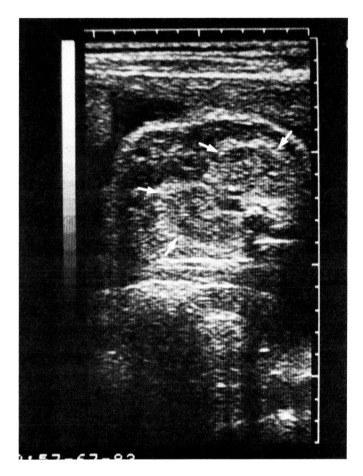

Fig 8-37. Polycystic renal dysplasia. Microscopic cysts of the collecting tubules characteristic of polycystic renal dysplasia produce enlarged kidneys with increased echogenicity (arrows).

collecting tubules result in increased echogenicity of these kidneys. Although the prenatal appearance of the complete lesion is fairly clear, early prenatal diagnosis is unsure, since cases of polycystic dysplasia have been reported that appeared normal early in pregnancy.

Renal agenesis results in a group of related clinical findings known as Potter's syndrome. Potter's syndrome includes renal agenesis, pulmonary hypoplasia, severe oligohydramnios, and compression malformations of the limbs and face and is uniformly fatal. Whenever severe oligohydramnios is discovered prior to 28 weeks' gestation, renal agenesis should be suspected. A careful sonographic examination of the fetal kidneys and bladder should be performed. Although a visible bladder is probable evidence of renal function, absence of a visible bladder must be confirmed by extended observation, since it is possible that the fetus had recently voided. Occasionally small bladders have been seen despite renal agenesis, presumably containing tissue transudate only. Furthermore, the adrenal hypertrophy commonly seen with renal agenesis might simulate kidneys on transverse scan. Maternal administration of a diuretic to stimulate fetal urine production during sonographic observation may be helpful after 24 weeks' gestation, but a reliable fetal response before that time is not ensured even with kidneys.

Ureterovesical Reflux

Mild, nonprogressive fetal hydronephrosis is seen with congenital ureterovesical reflux (Fig 8-38). In such a case, amniotic fluid volume should remain normal and the bladder is not enlarged. Mild hydronephrosis has been reported to resolve spontaneously during pregnancy, and documented congenital reflux can resolve later without treatment during infancy.

LONG BONE DYSPLASIAS

Fetal long bone length demonstrates a precise correlation to gestational age. A large variety of bone dysplasias cause an alteration of this growth. In many cases, the result is mild dwarfism. In other cases, notably thanatophoric dysplasia, the condition is fatal (Fig 8-39). Many of the types of long bone dysplasias that the sonographer might encounter in the fetus are summarized in Table 8-1. The diagnosis is based not only on bone length below the lower limit of normal for a given gestational age but also often on the shape of the bones and the size or shape of the fetal chest. Severe shortening of fetal long bones coupled with reduced chest size on transverse scan strongly suggests one of the severe fatal dysplasias. In the case of osteogenesis imperfecta, there are at least four types of affectation from very mild to lethal. Only in the case of the most severe types II and III is early prenatal diagnosis probable. Achondroplasia is the most common unexpected short limb condition in an infant born to normal parents, but it results in impairment of bone growth too mild to allow reliable prenatal diagnosis before 28 weeks' gestation.

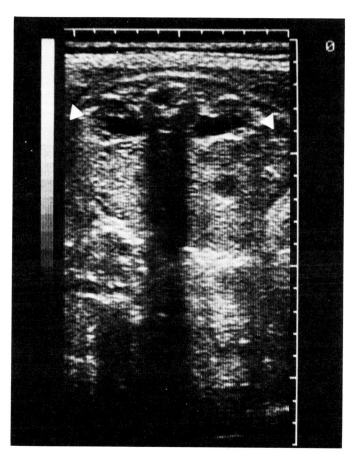

Fig 8-38. Ureterovesical reflux. Mild nonprogressive hydronephrosis may be the result of ureterovesical reflux. This transverse midabdominal scan demonstrates dilatation of the renal pelves. Solid triangles indicate outer margins of kidneys.

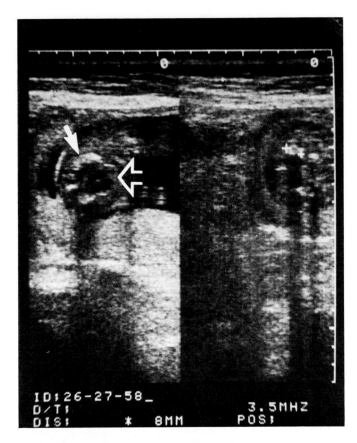

Fig 8-39. Thanatophoric dwarf. The right side of this sonogram demonstrates a shortened femur measuring 10 mm at 21 weeks'
gestation. On the left, the fetal heart (open arrow) is seen to
exceed the capacity of the fetal ribcage (solid arrow), strongly
suggesting the diagnosis of thanatophoric dwarf with severe
compromise of the fetal chest.

Whenever the fetal long bones are 6 mm or more below the expected
length for gestational age, a long bone dysplasia should be suspected. Mild
shortening may occur in an otherwise normal infant, however, and care
should be taken not to unnecessarily alarm the parents. Careful evaluation
of the fetal chest, methodical measurement of all long bones, and consultation with bone dysplasia experts may aid in defining the most probable
diagnosis.

Table 8-1. Prenatal Diagnosis of Long Bone Dysplasias

Type	Method	Gestational Age
Ellis-Van Creveld	Ultrasound	17 weeks
Campomelic	Ultrasound	21 weeks
Roberts' syndrome*	Ultrasound	22 weeks
Thanatophoric*	Ultrasound/x-ray	28 weeks
Diastrophic	Ultrasound/x-ray	18 weeks
Osteogenesis		
Type I	Ultrasound	20 weeks
Type II*	Ultrasound	19 weeks
Type III*	Ultrasound	19 weeks
Type IV	?	?
Hypophosphatasia	Ultrasound	14 weeks
Achondroplasia	Ultrasound	24 weeks

*Fatal

SUGGESTED READINGS

Asher JB, Sabbagha RE, Tamura RK, et al: Fetal pulmonary cyst: Intrauterine diagnosis and management. *Am J Obstet Gynecol* 151:97–98, 1985.

Aylsworth AS, Seeds JW, Guilford B, et al: Prenatal diagnosis of a severe deforming type of osteogenesis imperfecta. *Am J Med Genet* 19:707–714, 1984.

Baker ME, Rosenberg ER, Bowie JD, et al: Transient in utero hydronephrosis. *J Ultrasound Med* 4:51–53, 1985.

Blackwell DE, Spinnato JA, Hirsch G, et al: Antenatal ultrasound diagnosis of holoprosencephaly: A case report. *Am J Obstet Gynecol* 143:848–849, 1982.

Blumenthal DH, Rushovich AM, Williams RK, et al: Prenatal sonographic findings of meconium peritonitis with pathologic correlation. *J Clin Ultrasound* 10:350–352, 1982.

Callen PW, Bolding D, Filly RA, et al: Ultrasonographic evaluation of fetal paranephric pseudocysts. *J Ultrasound Med* 2:309–312, 1983.

Chervenak FA, Berkowitz RL, Romero R, et al: The diagnosis of fetal hydrocephalus. *Am J Obstet Gynecol* 147:703–716, 1983.

DeVore GR, Siassi B, Platt LD: The use of the abdominal circumference as a means of assessing m-mode ventricular dimensions during the second and third trimesters of pregnancy in the normal human fetus. *J Ultrasound Med* 4:175–182, 1985.

Dubbins PA, Kurtz AB, Wapner RJ, et al: Renal agenesis: Spectrum of in utero findings. *J Clin Ultrasound* 9:189–193, 1981.

Hadlock FP, Deter RL, Carpenter R, et al: Sonography of fetal urinary tract anomalies. *AJR* 137:261–267, 1981.

Henderson SC, Van Kolken RJ, Rahatzad M: Multicystic kidney with hydramnios. *J Clin Ultrasound* 8:249–250, 1980.

Hobbins JC, Bracken MB, Mahoney MJ: Diagnosis of fetal skeletal dysplasias with ultrasound. *Am J Obstet Gynecol* 142:306–312, 1982.

Holzgreve W, Curry CJR, Golbus MS, et al: Investigation of nonimmune hydrops fetalis. *Am J Obstet Gynecol* 150:805–812, 1984.

Kaitila I, Ammala P, Karjalainen O, et al: Early prenatal detection of diastrophic dysplasia. *Prenatal Diagnosis* 3:237–244, 1983.

Kurtz AB, Wapner RJ: Ultrasonographic diagnosis of second-trimester skeletal dysplasias: A prospective analysis in a high-risk population. *J Ultrasound Med* 2:99–106, 1983.

Lange IR, Manning FA: Antenatal diagnosis of congenital pleural effusions. *Am J Obstet Gynecol* 140:839–840, 1981.

Lee TG, Warren BH: Antenatal diagnosis of hydranencephaly by ultrasound: Correlation with ventriculography and computed tomography. *J Clin Ultrasound* 5:271–273, 1977.

Mahony BS, Callen PW, Filly RA, et al: Progression of infantile polycystic kidney disease in early pregnancy. *J Ultrasound Med* 3:277–279, 1984.

Mahony BS, Filly RA: High-resolution sonographic assessment of the fetal extremities. *J Ultrasound Med* 3:489–498, 1984.

Mayock DE, Hickok DE, Guthrie RD: Cystic meconium peritonitis associated with hydrops fetalis. *Am J Obstet Gynecol* 142:704–705, 1982.

Nikapota VLB, Loman C: Gray scale sonographic demonstration of fetal small-bowel atresia. *J Clin Ultrasound* 7:307–310, 1979.

Philipson EH, Wolfson RN, Kedia KR: Fetal hydronephrosis and polyhydramnios associated with vesico-ureteral reflux. *J Clin Ultrasound* 12:585–587, 1984.

Platt LD, Collea JV, Joseph DM: Transitory fetal ascites: An ultrasound diagnosis. *Am J Obstet Gynecol* 132:906–908, 1978.

Ray D, Berger N, Ensor R: Hydramnios in association with unilateral fetal hydronephrosis. *J Clin Ultrasound* 10:82–84, 1982.

Reilly KB, Rubin SP, Blanke BG, et al: Infantile polycystic kidney disease: A difficult antenatal diagnosis. *Am J Obstet Gynecol* 133:580–582, 1979.

Robinson HP, Hood VD, Adam AH, et al: Diagnostic ultrasound: Early detection of fetal neural tube defects. *Obstet Gynecol* 56:705, 1980.

Sabbagha RE, Tamura RK, Dal Compo S, et al: Fetal cranial and craniocervical masses: Ultrasound characteristics and differential diagnosis. *Am J Obstet Gynecol* 138:511–517, 1980.

Sanders R, Graham D: Twelve cases of hydronephrosis in utero diagnosed by ultrasonography. *J Ultrasound Med* 1:341–348, 1982.

Schaffer RM, Barone C, Friedman AP: The ultrasonographic spectrum of fetal omphalocele. *J Ultrasound Med* 2:219–222, 1983.

Shaff MI, Fleischer AC, Battino R, et al: Antenatal sonographic diagnosis of thanatophoric dysplasia. *J Clin Ultrasound* 8:363–365, 1980.

Wapner RJ, Kurtz AB, Ross RD, et al: Ultrasonographic parameters in the prenatal diagnosis of Meckel syndrome. *Obstet Gynecol* 57:388–391, 1981.

Young BK, Katz M, Klein SA: Intrapartum fetal cardiac arrhythmias. *Obstet Gynecol* 54:427–432, 1979.

Zemlyn S: Prenatal detection of esophageal atresia. *J Clin Ultrasound* 9:453–454, 1981.

Chapter 9

Sonography of the Placenta, Uterus, and Ovaries and of Ectopic Gestation

PLACENTA

Conditions of the placenta detectable with ultrasound include placenta previa, abruptio placentae, accessory lobes, and intraplacental hematomas. Transamniotic membranes may also be seen. Irregular vascular channels and a progressive increase in echogenicity within the placenta associated with aging may also be recognized with ultrasound.

Placenta Previa

The placenta may be low lying (Fig 9-1), the edge may extend over the internal os of the cervix (Fig 9-2), or the main body of the placenta may be placed directly over the os (Fig 9-3). Proper placental localization requires an accurate estimate of the location of the internal cervical os, which lies just below the bladder angle (Fig 9-4). Occasionally the cervical canal is discretely visible.

Apparent placental location can change as pregnancy progresses. A lower segment implantation or even apparent marginal previa found at scan before 20 weeks' gestation remains low lying in only about 7% of cases. Placenta previa is expected to occur in only about 3% of pregnancies in late gestation, and, therefore, the diagnosis of a low implantation early in gestation identifies a high-risk group deserving of later follow-up. Placental migration is often suggested to explain cases of apparent previa or low lying placentation noted early in gestation that are not low lying later. Actual placental movement is improbable. It is more likely that as the uterus grows, the location of the implantation site relative to the cervical os and lower segment shifts away in most cases. A clear central previa in early pregnancy is likely to remain a placenta previa.

159

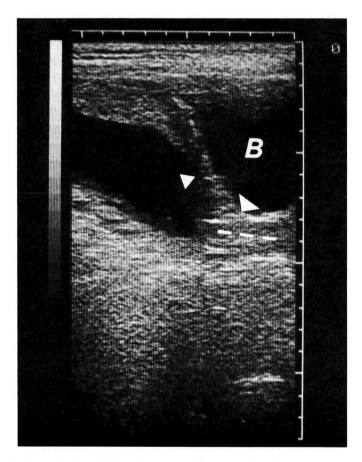

Fig 9-1. Anterior low lying placenta. The broad solid triangle indicates the bladder (B) angle and the expected location of the internal cervical os. The smaller solid triangle lies within the amniotic cavity and indicates the lowest margin of the placenta clearly separated from the internal os. The dashed line indicates the probable location of the endocervical canal.

Often it is difficult to identify precisely the edge of the placenta with respect to the internal os. The indistinct soft tissue echos originating from the vagina and portio of the cervix are easily lost in the mid pelvis. The bladder, therefore, helps to locate the cervical os. It is important that the patient be examined with a moderately full bladder whenever precise placental localization is desired, to allow proper localization of the internal

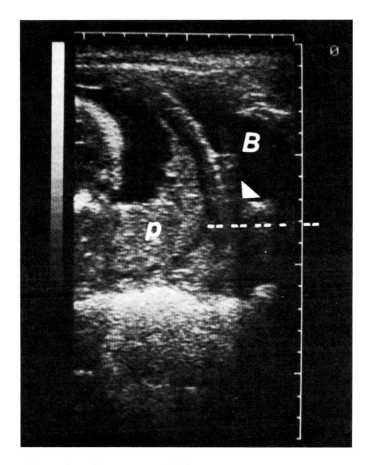

Fig 9-2. Posterior placenta previa. The solid triangle indicates the bladder angle and the probable location of the internal cervical os. The dashed line indicates the probable endocervical canal below the bladder (B). The placenta (p) extends from posterior up across the internal os, constituting a placenta previa.

cervical os. An overfilled bladder can confuse the location of the internal os as badly as an empty bladder.

Abruptio Placentae

Ultrasound is less reliable in its ability to confirm abruption of the placenta. Fresh clot demonstrates a diffuse echo pattern often closely

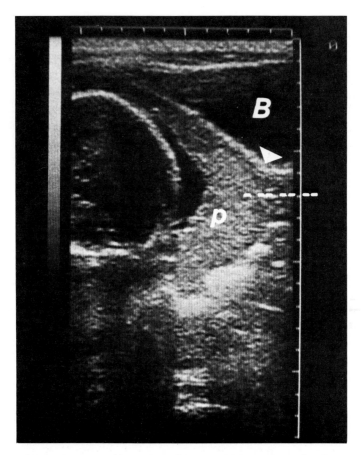

Fig 9-3. Central previa. Here the placenta (p) is seen to lie directly over the internal os of the cervix. The bladder (B) angle (solid triangle) indicates the position of the internal os, and the dashed line shows the probable location of the endocervical canal.

---

resembling placenta itself. This makes confident diagnosis of abruptio placentae difficult. Although with occasional dramatic examples the ultrasonic image might support such a diagnosis (Fig 9-5), in most cases sonography is not definitive and clinical judgment must predominate. Liquid blood, on the other hand, that might be found within a fresh intraplacental hematoma or lysed blood within an old hematoma would produce large echo-free areas within the substance of the placenta that are more clearly seen (Fig 9-6).

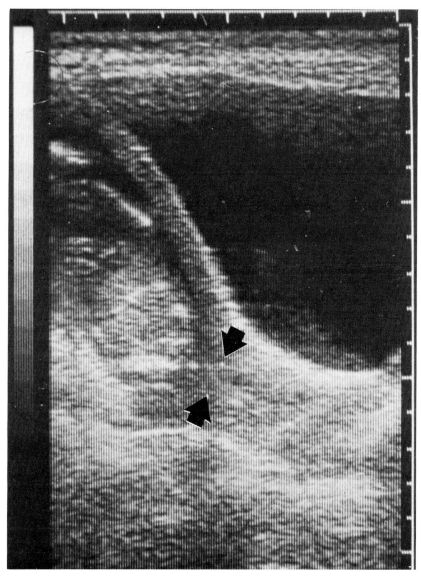

Fig 9-4. Proper placental location. This anterior lower midline scan of the pregnant uterus indicates the most probable location of the internal os of the cervix (arrows). It is here that measurements of the internal os may assist in the early diagnosis of premature dilatation of the internal os and incompetence of the cervix.

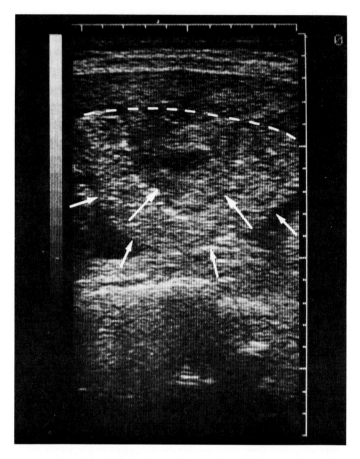

Fig 9-5. Abruptio placentae. This scan of the placenta of a fetus demonstrating some decelerations illustrates a fresh, echogenic blood clot elevating the central portion of the placenta. The clot (long arrows) may be differentiated by texture from the placenta (small arrows). The uterine margin is indicated by the dashed line. Delivery of this placenta shortly after this sonogram confirmed the composition of the central area as a blood clot.

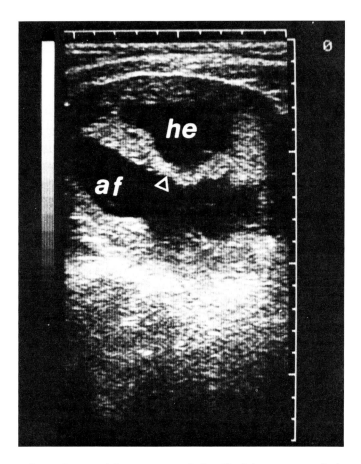

Fig 9-6. Intraplacental hematoma. A liquified hematoma (he) appears anechoic (black) similar to amniotic fluid (af) as illustrated here. The open triangle indicates the placenta.

Placental Texture

The differences in echo texture associated with aging probably relate to fibrin deposition within vascular channels. Echos originate from these surfaces, and, therefore, as fibrin deposition increases, echogenicity increases. Progression to calcification of these areas is associated strongly with fetal maturity.

Grade 0 is the least mature and is seen as the most homogeneous of placentas, with no peripheral cotyledonary echogenicity and a smooth chorionic plate. (The four grades are 0, I, II, and III.) A grade I placenta shows irregularities of the chorionic plate and anechoic (echo-free) areas under the chorionic plate and near the basilar plate (Fig 9-7). Grade II placentas have increased echogenicity incompletely surrounding the cotyledons but lack the shadowing that would suggest calcification (Fig 9-8). The peripheral echogenicity of the cotyledons is complete in a grade III placenta. There is calcification with shadowing, and there are typically central anechoic areas

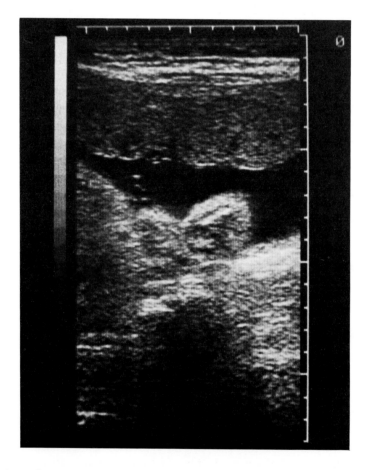

Fig 9-7. Grade I placenta. A grade I placenta has mild irregularities of the chorionic plate and some basilar echolucencies but little or no cotyledonary outlining and no calcifications.

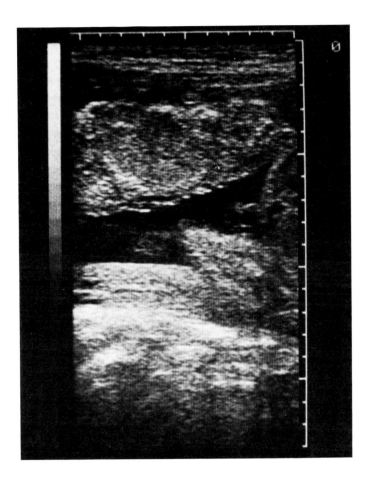

Fig 9-8. Grade II placenta. A grade II placenta has considerable echogenic outlining of the cotyledons. However, no calcifications and no shadowing are noted.

---

within the cotyledons (Fig 9-9). A placental grade is assigned on the basis of the most mature-appearing area.

Although there is correlation between grades of placental maturity and fetal pulmonary maturity, these visual data have not been shown to be sufficient evidence of maturity to justify elective delivery by itself. The risk is low that a fetus with a grade III placenta will develop serious respiratory distress, but a large number of mature fetuses have a lower grade of placenta.

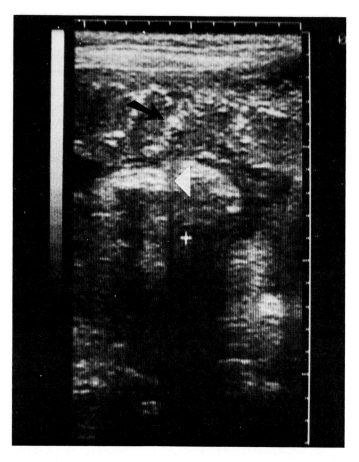

Fig 9-9. Grade III placenta. The calcifications (black arrow) casting acoustical shadows (solid triangle) are typical of the grade III placenta. Large and irregular venous lakes are frequently noted under the chorionic plate, and occasionally corpuscular flow may be noted on realtime ultrasound.

Vascular Channels

There is a wide variety to the size and shape of vascular channels visible in the placenta (Fig 9-10). Sometimes large basilar and subchorionic channels may be seen without serious clinical implications. Often, even corpuscular flow may be seen within these channels with realtime ultrasound.

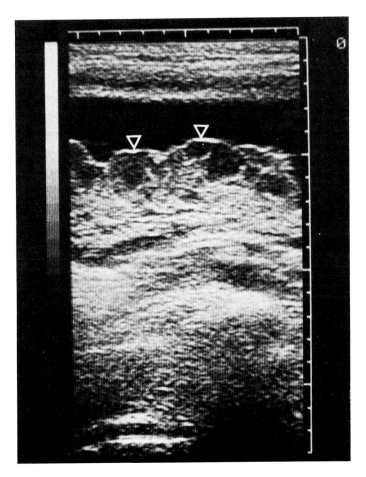

Fig 9-10. Vascular channels.

Amniotic Membranes

Transamniotic membranes may be seen with ultrasound, often originating from one margin of the placenta (Fig 9-11). Such membranes are of unclear significance and origin. Although perhaps analogous to amniotic bands, reported examples of membranes seen antenatally associated with fetal damage are rare. Such membranes might originate from delamination of the amnion or chorion after marginal bleeding. A hematoma might be cleared of red blood cells in time, leaving a seroma cavity bound by the delaminated membranes. Membranes might also remain from a nonviable twin.

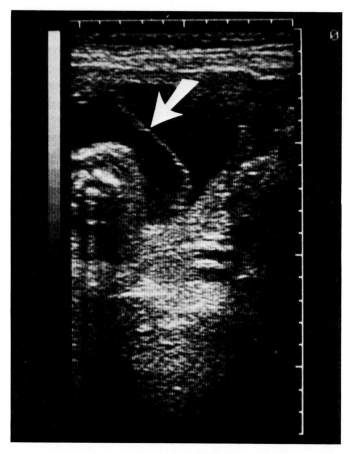

Fig 9-11. Intra-amniotic membranes. This echogenic membrane (arrow) was seen traversing the amniotic cavity of a singleton fetus. The demarcated extra cavity contained only fluid, and the pregnancy remained uncomplicated.

The finding of such membranes requires a careful search for possible fetal entanglement, but if none is found, no clear detrimental effect on the pregnancy can be predicted.

UTERUS

Uterine structural anomalies can be associated with repeated abortion, premature labor, or altered fetal growth and can occasionally be seen at scan. The uterus forms as the result of fusion in the midline of two paired müllerian primordia. Most uterine anomalies are the result of failure of complete midline fusion. Since fusion begins caudally and moves cranially, the spectrum of abnormalities ranges from the subseptate uterus to the didelphus with two separate cervices. Abnormalities that include duplication of the cervix may be diagnosed clinically, but those involving only the upper fundus require radiographic or ultrasonic studies. In the case of the subseptate uterus, the defect may result in persistent fetal malpresentation or premature labor (Fig 9-12). The gestation may fill the uterus, but deformation of the cavity is often apparent. With the bicornuate uterus, on the other hand, pregnancy is limited to one horn of the uterus and the hypertrophied nonpregnant horn is often seen to one side. The nonpregnant side presents a low-grade echo pattern with loosely organized internal structure typical of a mix of muscle and vascular channels. The decidual plate of the nonpregnant endometrial cavity is often seen as a hyperechogenic strip.

Leiomyomata uteri are common, usually benign muscle tumors of the uterus. These growths are often hormone responsive and may grow as pregnancy progresses. Leiomyomata may be located anywhere within the wall of the uterus or appear pedunculated from the serosal surface. In early pregnancy, patients often complain of abdominal pain, and even spotting. On scan, leiomyomata are seen to be well-circumscribed soft tissue masses of low-grade echogenicity with apparent but poorly organized internal structure (Fig 9-13). These masses may be small or quite large relative to the pregnancy and on occasion even represent an obstruction to vaginal delivery. Follow-up evaluations to track the growth of these tumors is often useful in clinical management. It is a common observation that placental implantation occurs over leiomyomata, perhaps because of increased vascularity.

THREATENED ABORTION AND ECTOPIC PREGNANCY

As early as 6 weeks' gestation a sac may be seen with realtime ultrasound, and by 8 weeks heart motion is usually seen. By 10 weeks, a fetal shape should be apparent, and significant fetal anatomy should be seen by 12 weeks. An early scan can significantly help clarify the prognosis of an early pregnancy by detecting deviation from these expected sonographic milestones.

Multiple investigators have reported that ultrasonic observation of a fetal mass with heart motion in the case of early bleeding is associated with retention of the pregnancy in most cases. The level of prognostic confidence of these sonographic findings exceeds any hormonal assay available. The positive predictive value of finding a fetus and a heartbeat in a pregnancy

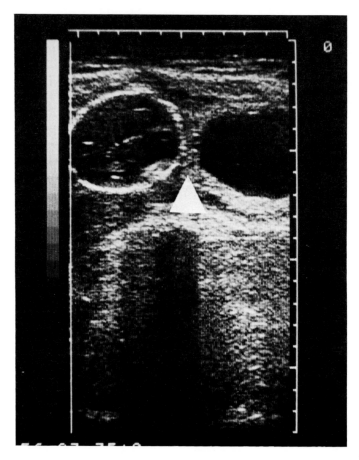

Fig 9-12. Subseptate uterus. This transverse scan of the fundus of a uterus at approximately 18 weeks' gestation illustrates the fetal cranium to the left side of a uterine septum (solid triangle). The amniotic fluid (black area) to the right side of the septum was confluent with the amniotic cavity of the fetus.

---

that is bleeding is not 100%, however, and the accuracy of the method should not be overrepresented to the patient. However, most patients are reassured by positive results.

The use of ultrasound in the care of the patient with a possible ectopic pregnancy is based on the ability to identify an intrauterine pregnancy and on the extreme rarity of a coexisting ectopic. In the patient with bleeding, abdominal pain, and unprotected intercourse, the finding of an intrauterine

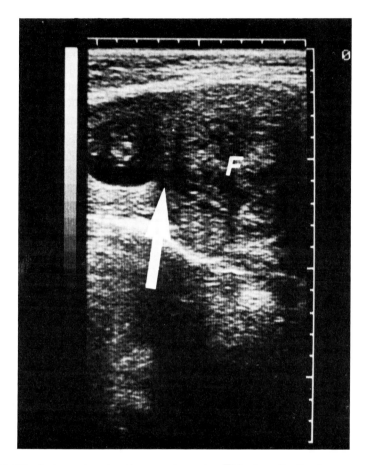

Fig 9-13. Leiomyomata plus pregnancy. This longitudinal scan of the pregnant uterus at approximately 8 weeks' gestation illustrates a large lower segment leiomyomata (F) with its typical disorganized soft tissue anatomy. The 8-week pregnancy is seen superior to the leiomyoma above the large arrow.

pregnancy indicates that she does not have an ectopic pregnancy. However, about 20% of patients with ectopic pregnancies demonstrate a sufficiently intense decidual reaction within the uterus to mimic a gestational sac on ultrasound. The anechoic (echo-free) cavity may be the result of trapped shed decidua or blood. For the sonographer to rule out an ectopic pregnancy, a gestational sac and a fetus must be seen and they must be clearly within the uterine cavity.

In exceptional instances, an ectopic pregnancy may be diagnosed when the fetus is found in the adnexae (Fig 9-14). This illustrates again the need to explore beyond the uterus when performing an ultrasound examination. In some cases, the information from a scan can be extended by simultaneously performing a pelvic examination. In some cases, manual manipulation of the uterus during ultrasonic observation can separate the uterus from the

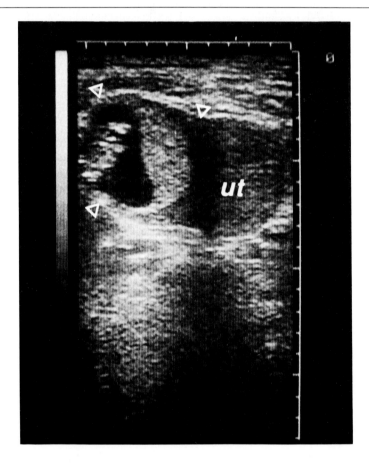

Fig 9-14. Cornual ectopic pregnancy. This transverse scan of the pregnant uterus at approximately 8 weeks' gestation illustrates a pregnancy eccentric to the right side of the uterus. The open triangles indicate a gestational sac extending from the right side of the uterus. The pregnancy and the uterus (ut) move together during pelvic examination, and soft tissues slide easily on the surface.

pregnancy. Insertion of a uterine sound into the cervical canal under ultrasonic observation can be necessary to establish the relationship of a pregnancy to the intrauterine cavity.

HYDATIDIFORM MOLE

Hydatidiform mole is a rare tumor of the trophoblast that on occasion can coexist with a fetus. In half of the cases the uterus is larger than expected for dates, while in the rest the uterus is normal size or even small for dates. Bleeding is a common presenting complaint, and on pelvic examination the ovaries are often enlarged.

The ultrasonic appearance of a molar pregnancy is unique. The uterus is filled with tissue of a relatively uniform echogenic texture (Fig 9-15). In comparison with leiomyomata, the tissue texture is more uniform and of greater echodensity. Examination of the ovaries often reveals bilateral multiple theca lutein cysts. An elevated quantitative serum human chorionic gonadotropin assay is confirmatory.

OVARIAN CYSTS

Examination of the adnexae is relatively easy with ultrasound; yet neglect of this important area is common (Fig 9-16). Although ovarian cysts persisting beyond the first trimester are uncommon, and the risk of malignancy is low, such tumors can never be ignored. Sonography in most cases is the easiest method of diagnosis and in many others is the only practical method of surveillance. These cystic masses may be characterized as to internal structure and followed for growth.

OTHER ADNEXAL FINDINGS

Other soft tissue masses may occupy the pelvis. Certainly, the existence of a pelvic kidney may not have been suspected prior to a patient's first pregnancy, and the clinical finding of such a large pelvic mass can be clarified with sonography. Furthermore, both maternal kidneys and the maternal gallbladder may be easily visualized with ultrasound and the status of renal obstruction or biliary disease evaluated by experienced observers. It is not suggested that obstetrical sonographers necessarily become experts at renal or gallbladder ultrasound, but they should be aware of the possibility of these applications and consider referral for such services if the clinical situation suggests disease.

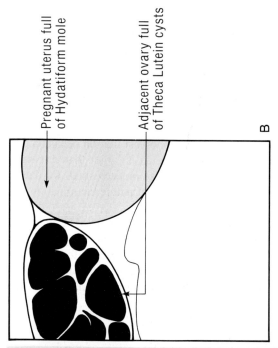

Pregnant uterus full
of Hydatiform mole

Adjacent ovary full
of Theca Lutein cysts

B

Fig 9-15. Hydatidiform mole. (*A* and *B*) Typical sonographic appearance of an intrauterine hydatidiform mole with multiple theca lutein cysts of the right ovary.

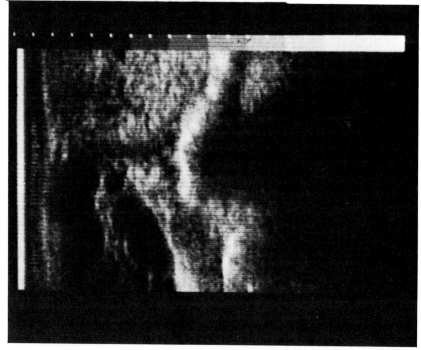

A

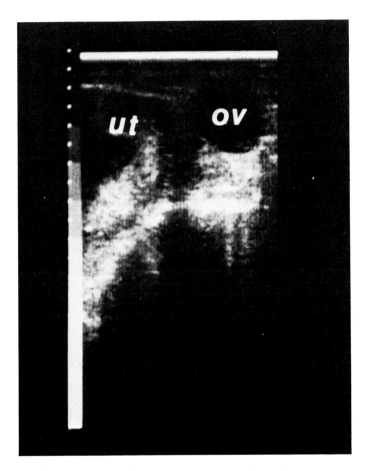

Fig 9-16. Ovarian cysts. Transverse scan of the left cornual area of a uterus (ut) at approximately 16 weeks' gestation illustrating a 2.5 to 3 cm ovarian cyst (ov) outside the uterus.

It is appropriate to emphasize the importance of adnexal scanning at every obstetrical ultrasound examination. It is too easy to view the uterine margins as the limits of an obstetrical scan and by doing so eliminate the possibility of making any of these diagnoses.

SUGGESTED READINGS

Ashton SS, Russo MP, Simon NV, et al: Relationship between grade III placentas and biparietal diameter determinations. *J Ultrasound Med* 2:127–129, 1983.

Bernstine RL, Lee SH, Crawford WL, et al: Sonographic evaluation of the incompetent cervix. *J Clin Ultrasound* 9:417–420, 1981.

Burrows PE, Lyons EA, Phillips HJ, et al: Intrauterine membranes: Sonographic findings and clinical significance. *J Clin Ultrasound* 10:1–8, 1982.

Cadkin AV, McAlpin J: The decidua-chorionic sac: A reliable sonographic indicator of intrauterine pregnancy prior to detection of a fetal pole. *J Ultrasound Med* 3:539–548, 1984.

Grannum PAT, Berkowitz RL, Hobbins JC: The ultrasonic changes in the maturing placenta and their relation to fetal pulmonic maturity. *Am J Obstet Gynecol* 133:915–922, 1979.

Hopper KD, Komppa GH, Bice P, et al: A reevaluation of placental grading and its clinical significance. *J Ultrasound Med* 3:261–266, 1984.

Nelson P, Bowie JD, Rosenberg ER: Early intrauterine pregnancy or decidual cast: An anatomic-sonographic approach. *J Ultrasound Med* 2:543–547, 1983.

Parulekar SG, Kiwi R: Ultrasound evaluation of sutures following cervical cerclage for incompetent cervix uteri. *J Ultrasound Med* 1:223–228, 1982.

Petrucha RA, Golde SH, Platt LD: Real-time ultrasound of the placenta in assessment of fetal pulmonic maturity. *Am J Obstet Gynecol* 142:463–467, 1982.

Smith C, Gregori CA, Breen JL: Ultrasonography in threatened abortion. *Obstet Gynecol* 51:173–177, 1978.

Chapter 10

Office Ultrasound: Setup

CHOICE OF EQUIPMENT

The selection of an ultrasound machine is the first major decision in the beginning of an office ultrasound service. First, the type of machine must be considered. Static, linear array, and mechanical sector scanners all have specific advantages and disadvantages. In addition, each brand of machine offers a variety of features to consider.

It is impractical for the obstetrician to consider the compound static type of machine for an office practice. Static machines are large, expensive, immobile, and incapable of assessing the dynamic features of a pregnancy such as fetal breathing movements that relate to fetal well-being. The choice, for an office practice, is between the linear array or the mechanical sector, or a combination of both.

Linear Array or Sector?

The image clarity between these two types of realtime machines does not differ substantially. Selection depends more on questions of versatility, format, and cost. The ideal machine configuration for one practice may not be ideal for another. Remember that the necessary contact area for a sector transducer is small and that this small area offers specific advantages in clinical applications that allow only limited surface access. Gynecological applications favor a sector machine. Imaging the organs of the nonpregnant pelvis is easier with a sector scanner because relatively minor changes in orientation of the transducer allow wide exploration of the pelvis from a limited suprapubic viewpoint. Therefore, if the projected use includes a large number of gynecological scans, either a sector or a machine with both linear and sector capabilities might be preferable to equipment limited to linear array alone.

The major disadvantage of a sector scanner for obstetrical applications is the limited near field of view. Beyond 24 weeks' gestation, it is difficult to include whole cranial or transverse fetal abdominal images in the field. Furthermore, in far advanced pregnancies the serious loss of image clarity in the far field of sector images is a detriment.

The linear array offers the obstetrician the best overall applicability if equipment selection is limited to a single type of machine. The field of view is rectangular, and there is wider near field capacity. Furthermore, although there is an inevitable loss of lateral resolution in the far field, there is no lateral motion artifact in the far field as is often apparent with sector scanners. It is, for many observers, easier to develop a sense of spatial orientation with the rectangular field of view of a linear array than with the wedge shape of the sector, but this is a minor consideration and with practice it is easily overcome. There are several brands that offer the option of both linear array and sector formats in the same piece of equipment. Although such a combination would seem to represent the ideal, this added versatility is expensive, and the added cost must be included in the cost analysis of the investment.

Brand Choices

There is a wide variety of specific brands to choose from with widely varied features. The cost also varies widely. The most important feature to evaluate when choosing an office scanner is image quality. Image quality is central to accurate measurements and sensitive evaluations of fetal anatomy. Clinical sonography is simplified if the choice of machine is governed by image quality first. It is very important to observe and personally work with a machine prior to purchase. It is best to work with a machine for several days to appreciate fully the image quality and other features.

Mechanical reliability, service support, and educational support from the vendor are also important factors to evaluate. Machine mobility may be important if movement of the equipment is a predictable necessity, but an attempt should be made to limit movement since it can adversely affect machine reliability. The cost of maintenance contracts that will be necessary after expiration of the warranty should also be considered at the time of initial purchase.

Last at all, consider the electronic gimmickry that has become popular in the field of ultrasound. Contemporary machines include pre-programmed gestational age readouts including biparietal diameter, femur length, and even abdominal circumference. Many of these microprocessor-based features will even average the estimated gestational age from multiple parameters and highlight any incompatible discrepancies. However, there are intrinsic disadvantages to being pre-committed to an arbitrarily selected growth curve or group of growth curves. As we have already discussed, any individual gestational age chart may not fit an individual practitioner's technique of measurement or the clinical population. Remember the discussion of interstudy variability in Chapter 4 and you will be immediately suspicious of equipment that ties you to one specific set of data. Furthermore, dependence on electronic aids may create a problem if the system breaks down. Alternative written charts must be kept available. Finally, extensive and complex electronic functions require considerable training to operate the equipment properly and might introduce the possibility of error from incorrect operation. Built-in gestational age charts are not necessarily bad, and most machines can be configured to suit a practice, but the potential hazards of being committed to a built-in age chart must be considered and anticipated before clinical or electronic problems arise.

The minimum necessary electronic functions are freeze-frame and electronic calipers. No currently available machine lacks these features. Other accessories that often prove useful are a Polaroid camera and a method of onscreen patient identification. Videotape capability and multiformat transparency cameras might be useful in teaching situations or if the clinician desires a method of recording, referral, and review of unusual ultrasound findings, but in most routine situations neither of these documentation techniques is clearly required.

OFFICE SPACE

Some attention to the selection of appropriate space early in the development of an office ultrasound service is necessary. The conversion of a typical examining room to an ultrasound room should be carefully considered. Often, family members are invited to observe a scan, and when the ultrasound is used to assist with amniocentesis, sufficient room for peripheral items such as tray, tables, and assistants should be provided. There ought to be easy access to a lavatory, and space for changing clothes should be available. The room should have a source of low intensity backlighting to optimize the visual qualities of the ultrasound machine.

Comfort and minimal distraction for the operator should guide the design and layout of the room. Although most scans can be performed while standing, fatigue is an insidious distraction, and a comfortable stool will minimize operator fatigue. Fatigue may cause the examiner to rush an ultrasound examination and might lead to inaccuracies or even missed diagnoses. Most right-handed operators prefer the patient table to their right side (Fig 10-1). The machine is then located to the left of the head of the table. Standing room might be provided to the patient's left for observers.

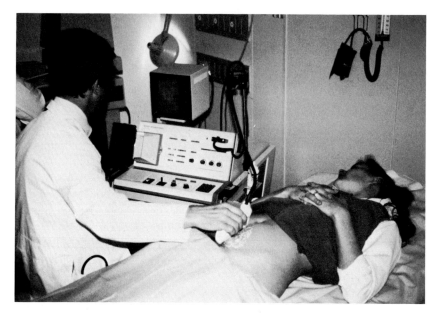

Fig 10-1. Ultrasound examining room. Appropriate arrangement of an ultrasound room for a right-handed examiner. The table and patient lie to the examiner's right and the ultrasound machine to his left, where both he and the patient can easily observe the scan. Both the patient and the examiner are comfortable, and there is an appropriate source of soft back-lighting.

CLINIC SCHEDULING

The composition and quality of a diagnostic ultrasound examination is often the result of subjective influences. Operator comfort and attitude are important in optimizing accuracy and sensitivity. Although it is not impossible to satisfy the need for accurate, sensitive sonography within the context of a busy prenatal clinic, this goal is more difficult when scanning sessions are randomly mixed with routine prenatal appointments. A busy schedule can be a distraction that influences the quality of ultrasonography. It is recommended at least in the beginning of an ultrasound service, that scans be done separately, allowing plenty of time for careful exploration in order to maximize both the learning experience and the results. After some confidence is developed, less time for the uncomplicated examination will be needed, but there is still considerable merit to structuring the clinic to provide nonemergent scanning appointments at a separate time from other clinical activities.

COST/REVENUE

In amortizing the investment cost of ultrasound equipment over 3 to 5 years it is appropriate to estimate that the usage will approximate one indicated scan for each delivery in an obstetrical practice. In arriving at an appropriate charge, the clinician must consider not only the cost of the equipment and maintenance but also the operator time. Overhead business costs are also necessary considerations. Each individual scan may be charged for, or cost recovery could be accomplished with general increment in an obstetrical package fee. The latter method eliminates a possible conflict of interests issue in the use of a diagnostic test from which the clinician benefits financially. A maximum sonography charge for those patients needing serial scanning would be reasonable.

Third party reimbursement varies both in amount and in the clinical indications for which reimbursement is allowed. The guidelines for reimbursement vary from area to area, and it is wise to consider local reimbursement guidelines when structuring a fee schedule for obstetrical ultrasound.

LIABILITY

Ultrasound is not immune to malpractice liability. Although there is no known direct risk of harm from the technique, inaccurate data or misdiagnoses can easily lead to inappropriate interventions and bad outcomes due to inadequate technique, experience, or equipment. Liability arises from failure to use the technique when indicated, as well as misuse of the technique. Litigation also results from the perception on the part of the patient that she has not received the service for which she paid. The limits of accuracy of ultrasound and the limits of resolution and diagnostic ability that may be obvious to the medical community are not always obvious to the patient. It is in the best interests of every sonographer to ensure that every patient is made aware of the reasonable limitations of ultrasound in the exact context of her examination. The patient should understand the clinical indications and the clinical goals for her examination. Each patient should be aware that an apparently normal ultrasound examination does not guarantee the birth of a perfectly normal child. In the opinion of many authorities it is appropriate to have the patient sign a permit that spells out these limitations in order to avoid any misconceptions. No such written document is perfect protection, but some written disclaimer may help to inform the patient more completely and more reliably than would otherwise be the case.

There is no consensus on the extent to which the office practitioner is obligated to record and retain documentation of each ultrasound examination. Actual practice varies from simple chart notes to extensive videotaping and multiformat photography of each examination. Documentation is certainly no protection against liability for error. Extensive photographic documentation can be useful as a learning tool if outcome does not confirm earlier sonographic results, but photographic documentation of an error would not be a helpful defense against litigation. Permanent photographs that do not reveal a missed malformation will not alter the reality of the unexpected birth of the malformed child.

It is clearly necessary to record the dimensional data from each sonographic examination in the patient's chart. Such a note should mention important features of the examination such as fetal number, position, placental location, amniotic fluid volume, fetal movements, and those areas of fetal anatomy that were evaluated. Fetal dimensions and the estimated gestational age from each dimension should also be included. A dedicated office form would encourage the operator to perform a complete examination each time. It would also be useful for the operator to maintain a log of examination with both clinical gestational age and ultrasonic dimensions to allow later analysis of technical accuracy at appropriate intervals. Polaroid or other types of photographs may be taken of unusual findings and also of those images on which clinical management will be based, such as biparietal diameter. More extensive documentation is expensive and is not likely to be productive in an office setting unless for teaching or consultation and referral purposes.

The subject of documentation of operator skills and training also remains unsettled. No recognized national examination currently exists for physicians performing ultrasound outside of board certification examinations in radiology and obstetrics/gynecology. No specified training requirements exist outside of residency or fellowship experience. On-the-job experience and postgraduate courses and mini-fellowships are the practical reality of post-residency training in obstetrical ultrasound. This is a reasonable and appropriate method of skill acquisition if careful clinical judgment is used in interpreting early results and incorporating them into patient care. Extreme care must be used when nonphysician office personnel are expected to perform ultrasound. Final responsibility and liability for such services are the physician's. Many states examine and register nonphysician sonographers and, therefore, the use of a nonregistered nonphysician in such a state might increase liability risks. Paramedical sonographers can save time and produce high quality results, but registration and certification is recommended when available, and close supervision by a physician is important both to quality patient care and to limitation of liability risks.

CONSULTATION

Ultrasound does not differ from any other clinical procedure in which appropriate consultation and referral is important to high quality results. Each operator brings to the examination a unique degree of skill and experience. For the usual patient in need of gestational age confirmation or placental localization, a detailed malformation evaluation or intrauterine weight estimation may not be clinically indicated. In the case of pregnancies at risk for a malformation, and in those cases in which malformation is suspected, referral resources should be clearly identified and available to allow easy consultation and review. Consultation can also be important in the case of significant measurement discrepancies. Tertiary referral for ultrasound examination can not only maximize the quality of patient care but also represent an important learning resource.

SUGGESTED READINGS

Anderson SG: Real-time sonography in obstetrics. *Obstet Gynecol* 51:284–287, 1978.

Perone N, Carpenter RJ, Robertson JA: Legal liability in the use of ultrasound by office-based obstetricians. *Am J Obstet Gynecol* 159:801–804, 1984.

Wetrich DW: Routine ultrasound scanning in midpregnancy. *Obstet Gynecol* 60:309–313, 1982.

Index

A

Abdominal anatomy, 37, 39–43, *44, 45, 46*
  See also Thoracoabdominal
    malformations
Abdominal circumference
  femur length relationship to, 75, *76,* 77
  fetal growth evaluation, 71–72
  fetal weight estimation, 73, 80, 81, 82, 83–84
  gestational age assignment, 62–64, *65, 66*
  head diameter ratios and, *72*
  intrauterine growth retardation
    diagnosis, 77
  mean head diameter and, 74–75
  See also Mean abdominal diameter
Abdominal lesions
  hydramnios and, 93
  See also Thoracoabdominal
    malformations
Abortion. *See* Miscarriage
Abruptio placentae, 161–162, *164, 165*
Achondroplasia, *157*
Acoustical impedance, 6
Acoustical shadows, 60
Adnexal examination, 175, 177
Adrenal hypertrophy, 154

Age. *See* Gestational age; Maternal age;
  Paternal age
Altitude, 49
Amniocentesis
  office space and, 181
  risk in, 87, 88
Amniotic fluid
  chest anatomy, *36*
  renal dysplasia, 152–153
  serum alpha-fetoprotein, 93
Amniotic fluid volume
  biophysical profile evaluation scoring, *76, 77*
  fetal growth evaluation, 73
  fundal height discrepancies and, 90
  gestational age and, 75
  intrauterine growth retardation
    diagnosis, 77
  prenatal diagnosis indications, 90–93
  ureterovesical reflux and, 154
Amniotic membranes, 169–170
A-mode, *8*
Amplitude
  echo and, *7*
  reflection and, *7*
  sound beams, 6
Anatomy. *See* Normal anatomy
Anencephaly
  gestational age, 29
  sonographic appearance of, 97, *98, 99*

Note: Folio references in italic type refer to figures, tables, and illustrations.

Aneuploidy. *See* Fetal aneuploidy
Angle movement
  illustrated, *26*
  uses of, 24
Animal studies, 19–20
Anterior horns of choroid plexes
  hydrocephalus and, 106, *109*
  See also Choroid plexes
Anterior horns of lateral ventricles,
  29–30, *31*
Anterior low lying placenta, *160*
Anthropomorphic asymmetry, 80
Aorta, 37, *39*
Aortic arch, 37, *39*
Aortic valvular atresia, 115, 121
Aqueductal stenosis, 103, 106
Arrhythmias. *See* Cardiac arrhythmias
Ascites
  cardiac malformations and, 121
  posterior urethral valve obstruction,
    144, *149*
  sonographic appearance of, *142,* 143
Atria (heart)
  malformations of, 121, *122, 123*
  normal anatomy, *36,* 37
Attenuation. *See* Dissipation
Automatic time gain, 11–12
Autosomal translocation, 89
Axial resolution, 14–*15*

B

Basilar plate, 166
Beam width
  electronic focusing and, *13*
  lateral resolution and, 12–13
  third dimension, 14
Bicornuate uterus, 171
Bilateral hydronephrosis, 144, *148*
Biliary disease (maternal), 175
Biophysical profile, *76,* 77
Biparietal diameter (BPD)
  femur length and, 64–65
  fetal growth impairment and, 71
  fetal weight estimation and, 73, 80,

    81, 82–83
  gestational age assignment and, 50–58
  illustration of, *56*
  interval growth rates and, 74–75
Birth asphyxia, 69
Birth defects
  acute clinical indications, 89–90
  amniotic fluid abnormalities, 92–93
  craniospinal malformations, 97–115
  etiological factors in, 88
  long bone dysplasias, 154–157
  thoracoabdominal malformations,
    115, 121–143
  ultrasound and, 95
  urinary tract abnormalities, 143–154,
    155
  See also Craniospinal malformations;
    Thoracoabdominal malformations;
    Urinary tract abnormalities; *entries*
    under names of specific birth
    defects and abnormalities
Birth method, 79–80
Birth weight
  amniotic fluid volume and, 73
  fetal growth evaluation and, 69
  prediction of, 80
  See also Fetal weight estimation
Bladder. *See* Gallbladder; Urinary
  bladder
B-mode, 9
Bone dysplasia. *See* Long bone
  dysplasias
Bowel
  cloacal plate anomalies and, 144, *151*
  perforation of, 135, *140, 141*
BPD. *See* Biparietal diameter (BPD)
Brachycephaly, 56
Bradycardia
  heart defects, 115, 121, *122, 123*
  prenatal diagnosis, 93
  See also Cardiac arrhythmias
Brain. *See* Craniospinal anatomy
Brain imaging, 16
Brain stem, 30, *32*
Breech presentation
  anencephaly and, 97